HIGH PROTEIN
RECIPE BOOK

High Protein Easy To Make Recipes

JULIA CAMMOILE

Copyright © 2019 by Julia Cammoile

All rights reserved. No part of this book may be used or reproduced by any means, graphic, electronic, or mechanical, including photocopying, recording, taping, or by any information storage retrieval system, without the written permission of the publisher except in the case of brief quotations embodied in critical articles and reviews.

WELCOME!

There are some cool features in this recipe book that will make it easy for you to cook the dishes and also track your food.

TRACKING YOUR FOOD

If you want to keep track of your macronutrients and calories, then all you have to do is scan the barcode on each recipe in your MyFitnessPal™ App and voila.

MEDICAL DISCLAIMER

This recipe book is not designed to replace any advice given to you by a medical practitioner or registered dietician.

All recipes within this book are for information purposes only. If you choose to make a recipe within this book, then you are doing so at your own risk. Please check all the ingredients first to ensure you are not allergic to any of them.

If you think there is any part of the book that might have a negative impact on your health, then please consult a doctor before starting.

Table of Contents

Eggs Royale 1

Breakfast Muffins.. 3

Apple & Cinnamon Slow Cooked Oats 5

Avocado Egg Nests... 7

Banana And Blueberry Protein Pancakes 9

Smoked Salmon And Sweet Potato Rosti 11

Dark Chocolate Overnight Oats 13

Tomato Egg Nests 15

Breakfast Smoothie 17

Avocado, Bacon & Egg On Toast 19

Chicken & Sweet Potato Hash 21

Chicken, Parma Ham, Avocado & Feta Salad... 23

Stuffed Peppers.. 25

Orange & Oregano Chicken Salad... 27

Chinese Spiced Duck Salad 29

Chilli Chicken And Avocado Wrap... 31

Ginger & Spring Onion Steamed Cod... 33

Chicken Stir Fry 35

Steak Salad 37

Hasselback Fajita Chicken... 39

Cod & Roasted Vegetables 41

EGGS ROYALE

(Per Serving) Calories 390 / Carbs 18g / Protein 30g / Fat 22g

For a simple yet sophisticated breakfast, brunch or lunch, you can't beat Eggs Royale. Buttery avocado goes so well with the silky smooth smoked salmon and a perfectly poached egg. Great for helping you to build muscle and lose weight

Serves 2 Prep Time 5 mins Cook Time 5 mins **INGREDIENTS** 2 Wholegrain Seeded Bread Slices Pinch of Salt 1 tsp Vinegar 4 Medium Eggs 1 Avocado 100g (3 1/2oz) Smoked Salmon	**HOW TO COOK IT** Put the water on the heat and bring to the boil. Place the bread in the toaster and toast. Add a pinch of salt and a tsp of vinegar to the boiling water. Create a swirl in the water and then quickly crack the eggs, add them to the water. Cook the eggs for 90 to 120 secs then remove from the water. Halve the avocado, remove the stone and mash both halves of the avocado. Spread the mashed avocado over both slices of toast. Place the smoked salmon on top of the avocado. Place the cooked eggs on top of the salmon and serve.

DIETICIAN'S NOTES

Higher protein breakfasts (25-30 grams of protein) are a great choice if your goal is weight loss, as they stave off hunger for longer than cereal based meals.

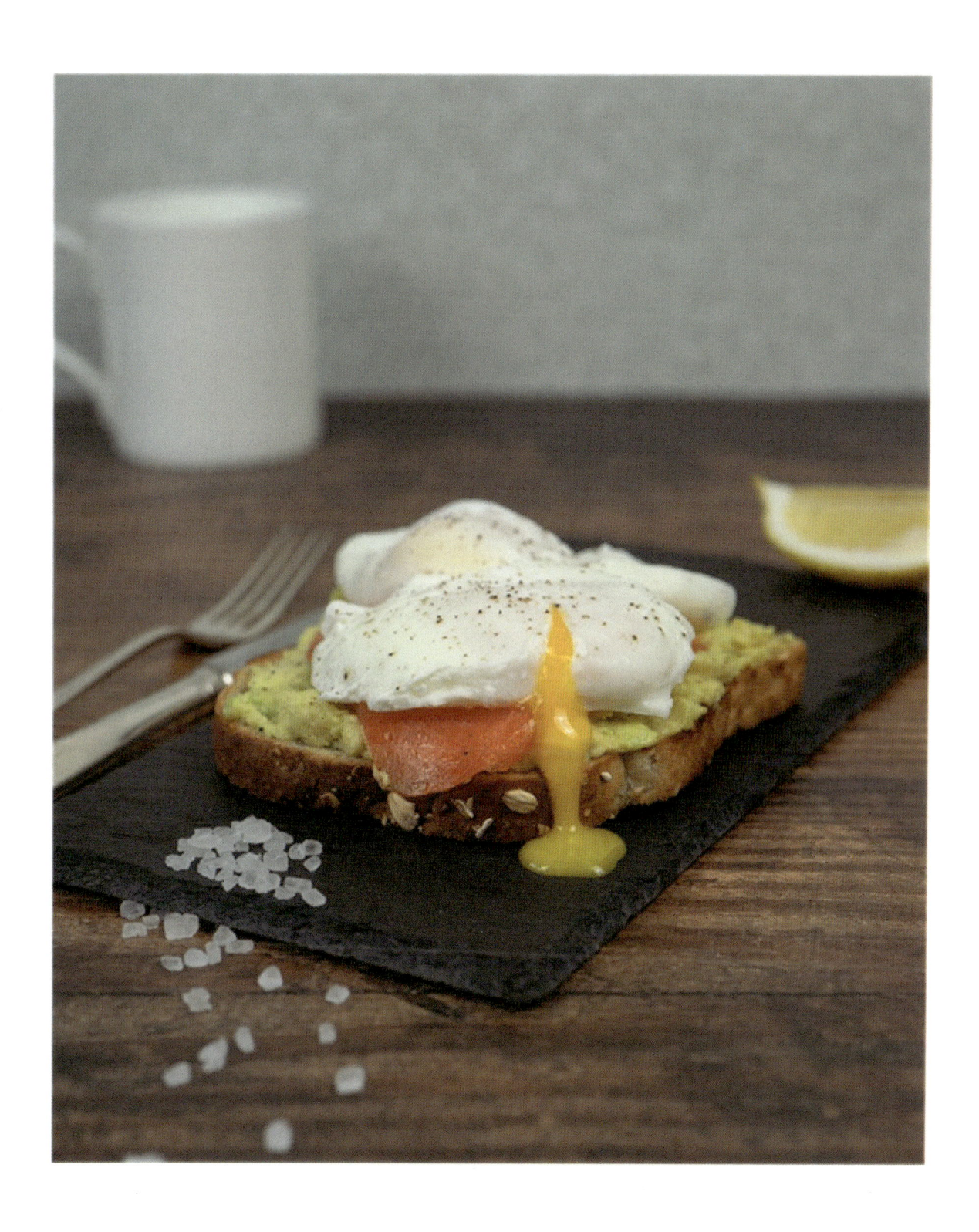

BREAKFAST MUFFINS

(Per Serving) Calories 329 / Carbs 7g / Protein 28g / Fat 21g

Ditch that egg and bacon McMuffin and make a healthy version instead! Red pepper and feta cheese add flavour and texture to these tasty breakfast muffins. This is an easy grab-and-go option for busy mornings!

| Serves 2 (3 muffins per person) Prep Time 10 mins Cook Time 25 mins

INGREDIENTS

6 Medium Eggs
Pinch of Pepper
2 Bacon Medallions
½ Onion
(finely chopped)
½ Red Bell Pepper (finely chopped)
50g (1 3/4oz) Feta Cheese (roughly chopped) | ## HOW TO COOK IT

Preheat oven to 200°C (400°F).

Crack the eggs into a mixing bowl, add pepper and whisk.

Grill the bacon on both sides until cooked, then cut into pieces.

Evenly distribute the onion, pepper and bacon into a muffin tin. I use a silicone muffin tin as the muffins are easier to remove afterwards.

Then pour the eggs into the muffin tin, aiming for an equal amount for each muffin.

Sprinkle the feta over the egg mixture.

Cook for 22 - 25 minutes.

When done, plate up or add to a tupperware container and take to work. |

DIETICIAN'S NOTES

Egg based breakfasts lower hunger hormones more effectively than cereal or toast, making them a smart choice if your goal is weight loss. Add chopped fresh herbs for an extra antioxidant boost.

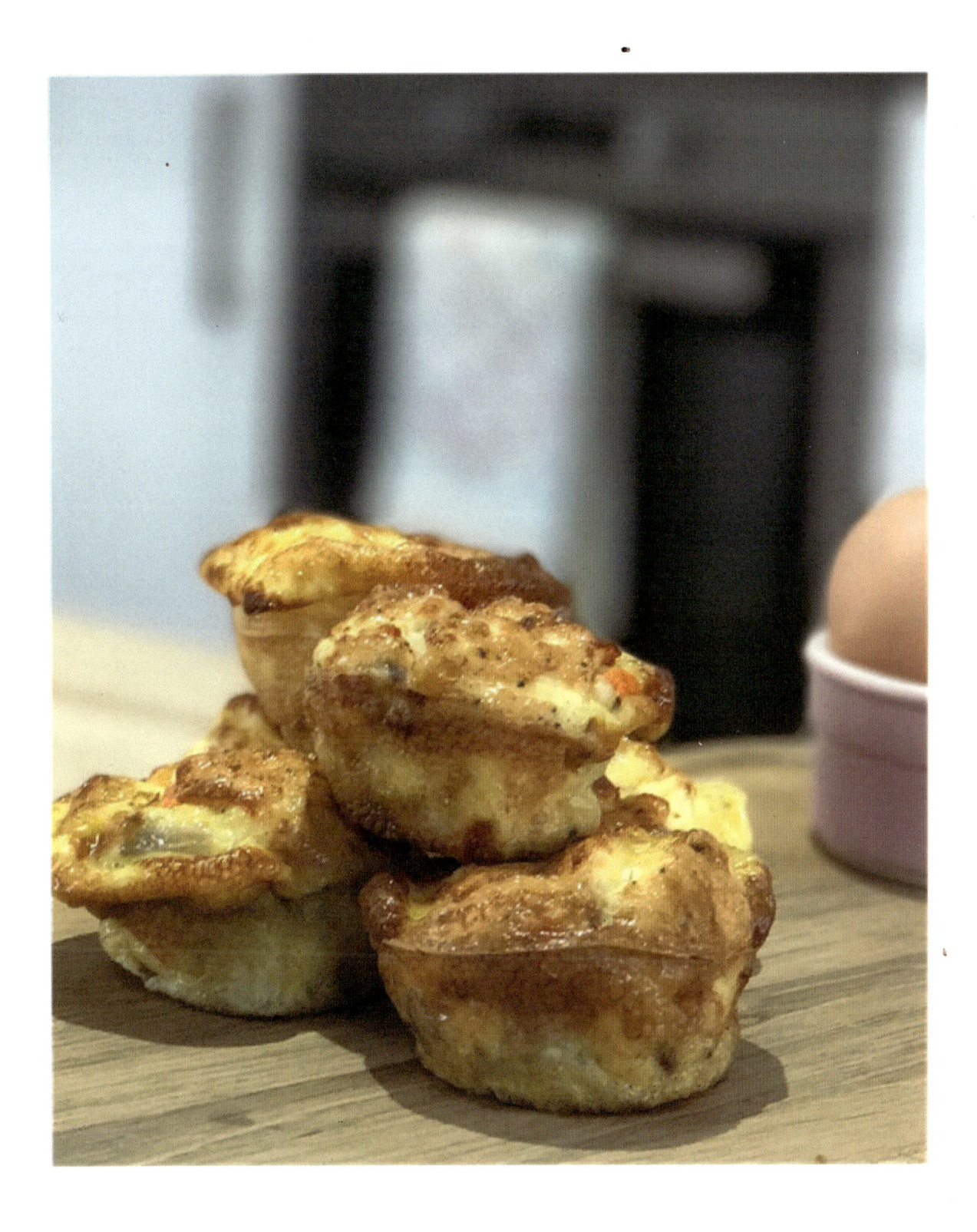

APPLE & CINNAMON SLOW COOKED OATS

(Per Serving) Calories 201 / Carbs 30g / Protein 9g / Fat 5g

This is a healthy, tasty breakfast that's warm, creamy, and slightly sweet with tender pieces of apple and plenty of cinnamon. Pop all of the ingredients in your slow cooker overnight and in the morning you'll wake up to a delicious, hearty breakfast.

| Serves 2
Prep Time 2 mins Cook Time 7 ½ hours

INGREDIENTS

45g (1 1/2oz) Porridge Oats
1 tsp Cinnamon
1 tsp White or Brown Sugar
350ml (1 1/2cups) Semi Skimmed Milk
1 Apple
(peeled, core removed and roughly chopped) | **HOW TO COOK IT**

Add the oats, cinnamon, and sugar to a glass bowl and mix.
Then add in the milk and stir well.
Finally add the apple into the glass bowl and quickly stir.
Fill the slow cooker bowl with cold water and then place the oat mixture in the glass bowl into the slow cooker.
Cook for 7 ½ hours on low then tuck in!
Optional: Add a sprinkle of cinnamon when done for extra flavour. |

DIETICIAN'S NOTES

Cinnamon is something of a secret weapon - it helps to slow down the absoprtion of carbohydrates, which may help regulate blood glucose levels. It's also a helpful source of antioxidants.

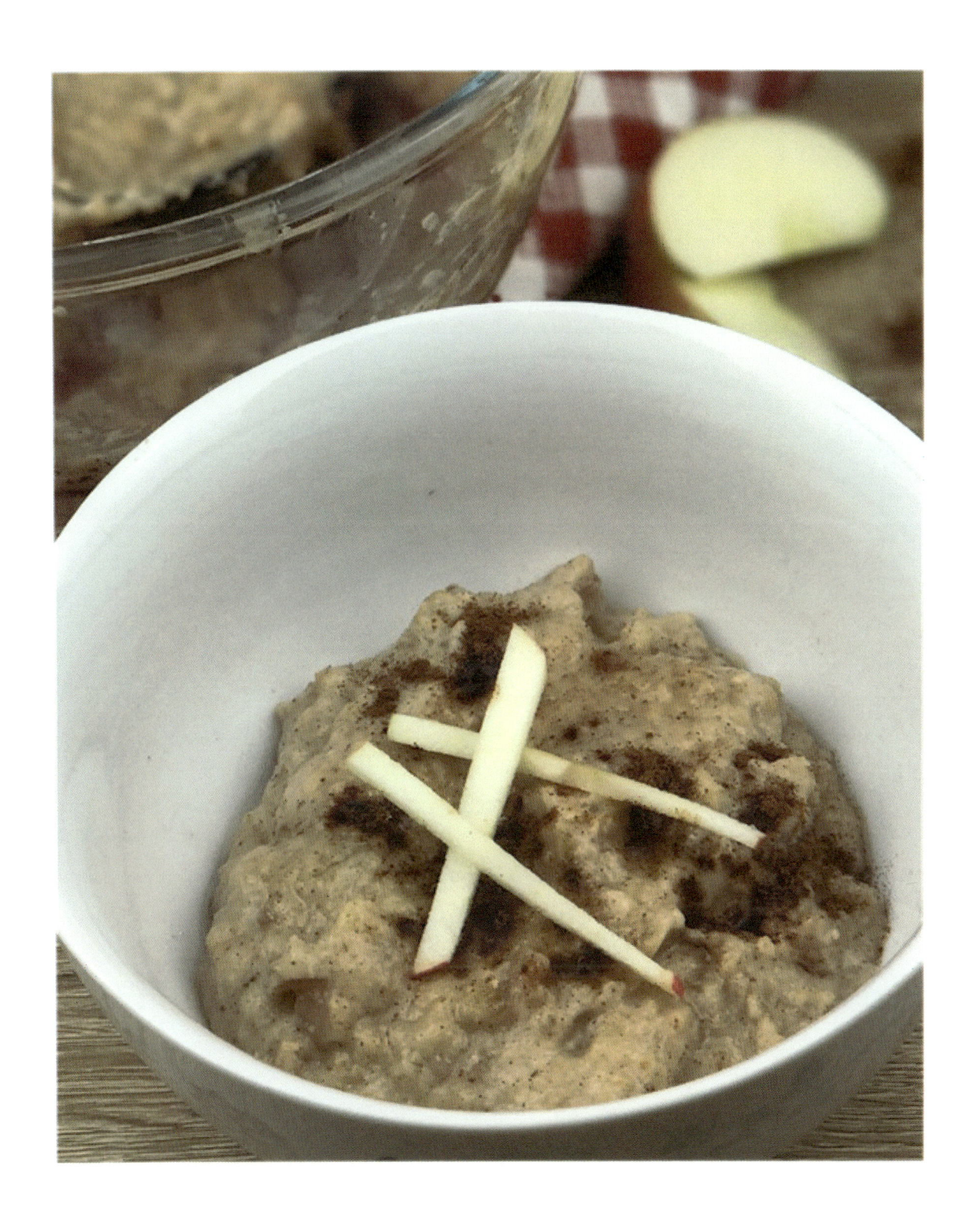

AVOCADO EGG NESTS

(Per Serving) Calories 629 / Carbs 18g / Protein 29g / Fat 49g

If you're a bit bored of the usual ways to have eggs, these quick-to-make nests will make eggs exciting again! Bake them in scooped out avocados, sprinkle on some feta and serve with juicy parma ham for a brunch or lunch with a difference!

Serves 1 Prep Time 5 mins Cook Time 20 mins **INGREDIENTS** 1 Large Avocado 2 Medium Eggs 20g (3/4oz) Feta Cheese 2 Slices Parma Ham	**HOW TO COOK IT** Preheat the oven to 200oC. Cut the avocado in half lengthways and remove the stone. Depending on the size of the holes, you may need to carve a slightly bigger hole. Cut a thin section off the avocado so it stands flat (see video). Place both halves on a baking tray. Separate the yolks and the egg whites. Put the yolks into the holes of the avocado and fill the rest of the hole with the remaining egg whites until full. Chop up the feta cheese and sprinkle on top of the avocado. Place in the preheated oven for 20 minutes. Leave to stand for 3 minutes. Plate up the Parma ham and tuck in! Tip: Too high in caloreis for you? Share this dish with someone to halve the calories!

DIETICIAN'S NOTES

Studies show the fibre and fats in avocados can help to regulate cholesterol levels. For an extra heart heathy dish, swap parma ham for a slice of omega-3 rich smoked salmon, and add a side of vegetables.

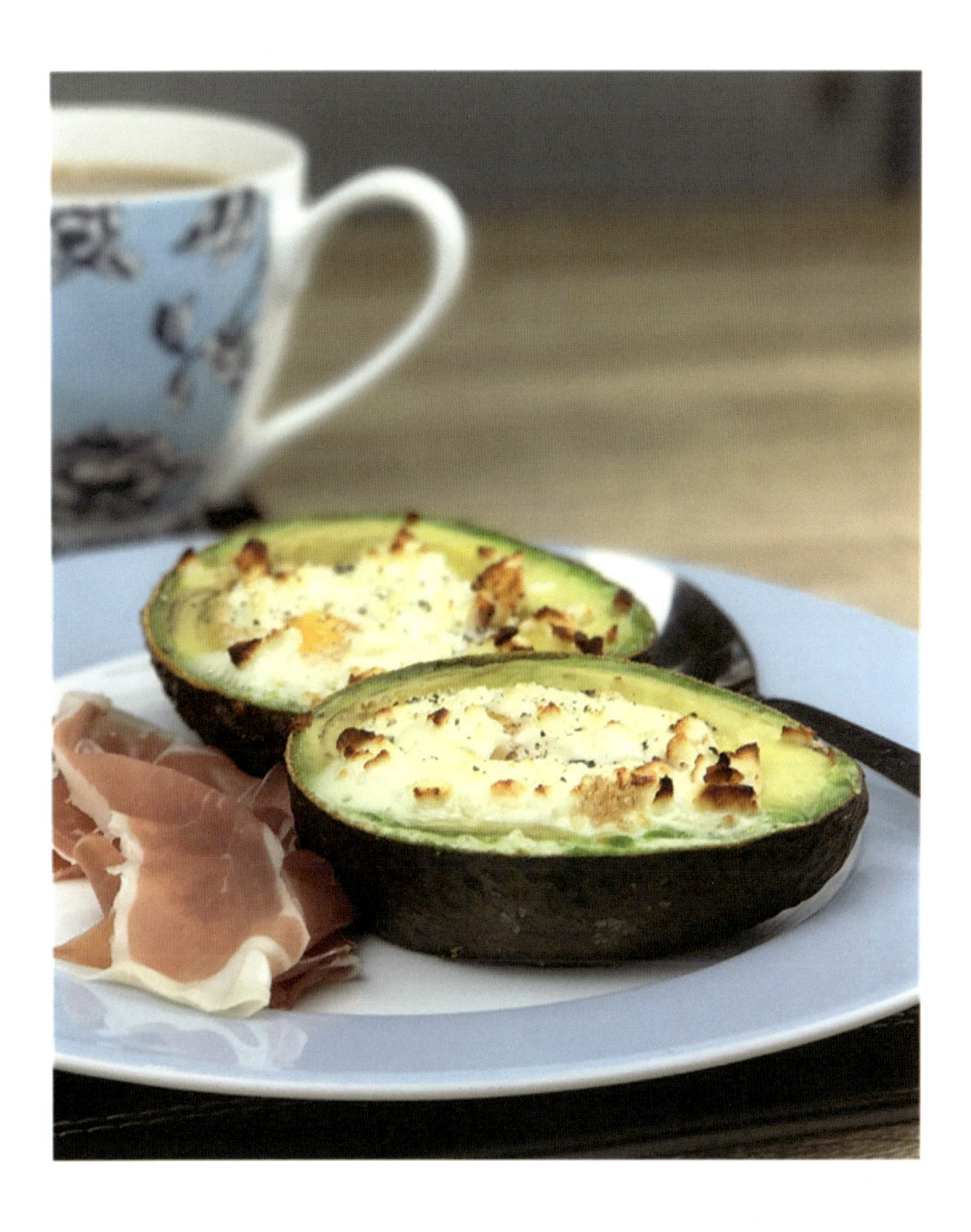

BANANA AND BLUEBERRY PROTEIN PANCAKES

(Per Serving) Calories 448 / Carbs 54g / Protein 31g / Fat 12g

These fruity pancakes are not only a brunch and breakfast favourite, but make a delicious dessert too, which should keep you feeling satisfied, thanks to the protein-packed ingredients. They are super-speedy and can be made in just twenty minutes!

| Serves 1
Prep Time 10 mins Cook Time 10 mins

INGREDIENTS

40g (1 1/2oz) Oats
25g (1oz) Chocolate Whey Protein
½ tsp Baking Powder
2/3 Banana
1 Medium Egg White
2 squares 70% Dark Chocolate
30g (1oz) Blueberries
30g (1oz) Greek Yogurt | ## HOW TO COOK IT

Put the oats in a blender and blend.
Then add protein powder, baking powder, half the banana and the egg white. Blend until it's all mixed together.
Put a bowl over boiling water and melt the chocolate.
Heat a frying pan over a medium heat then add half the mixture, place some blueberries on top and push them in.
Cook for 1 minute per side and then plate up.
Spoon the Greek yogurt on top of the pancakes along with the last of the banana and the blueberries.
Lastly, drizzle the melted dark chocolate over the pancakes and serve. |

DIETICIAN'S NOTES

Whey protein is rich in leucine, a protein buidling block which helps the body manufacture new muscle. Teamed with carbohydrate rich oats and banana, this would be a good choice pre or post workout.

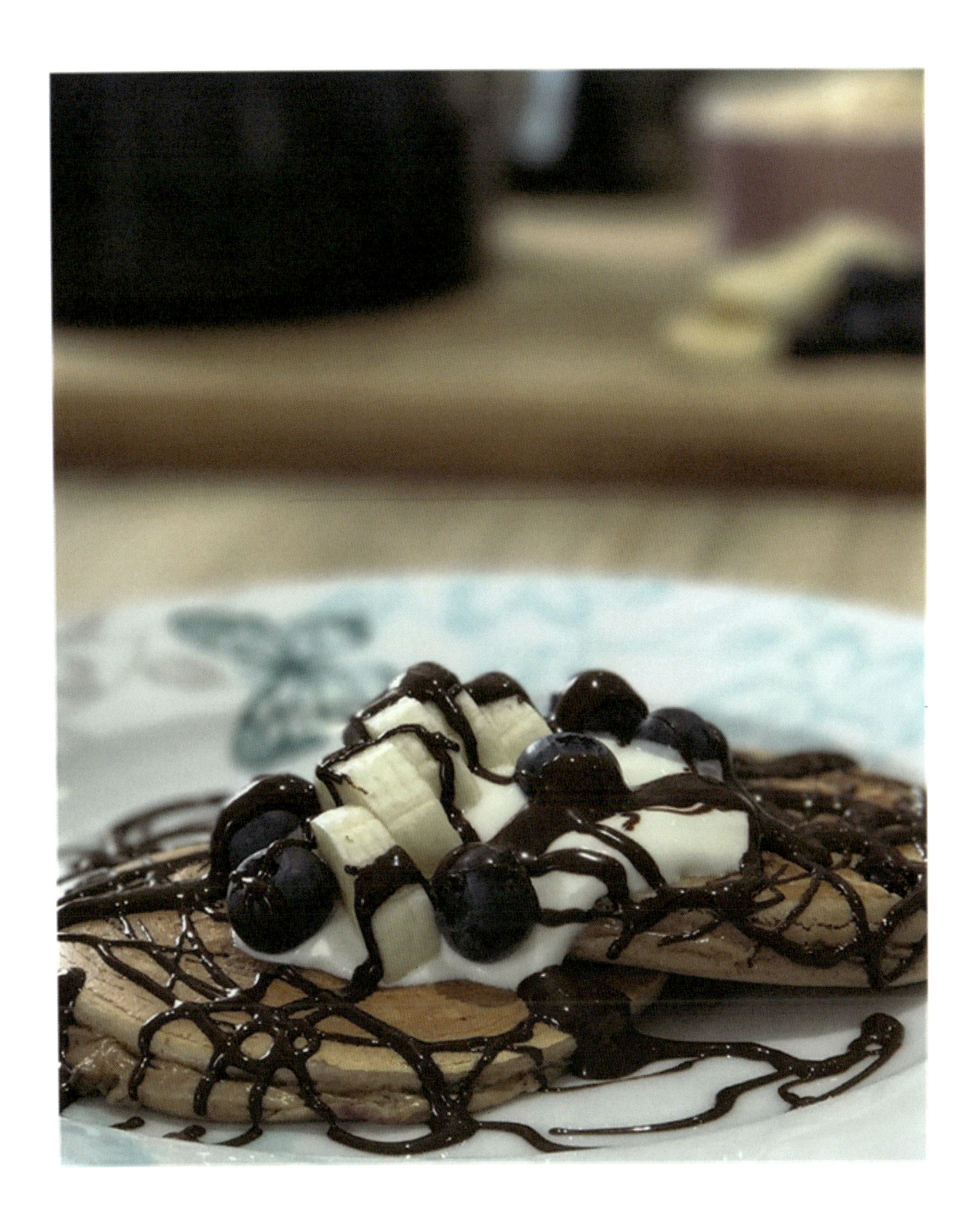

SMOKED SALMON AND SWEET POTATO ROSTI

(Per Serving) Calories 414 / Carbs 20g / Protein 34g / Fat 22g

Rosti are the Swiss version of hash browns, and using sweet potato gives them a delicious, crispy texture which goes really well with the poached eggs and creamy smoked salmon. This is a great choice for a weekend lunch or brunch!

Serves 1 Prep Time 10 mins Cook Time 5 mins ## INGREDIENTS 60g (2oz) Carrot (peeled and grated) 60g (2oz) Onion (peeled and grated) 50g (1 3/4oz) Sweet Potato (peeled and grated) 2 Small Eggs Pinch of Salt & Pepper 1 tsp Olive Oil 1 tsp Vinegar 100g (3 1/2oz) Smoked Salmon Lemon Wedge (cut into wedges)	## HOW TO COOK IT Peel the carrot, onion and sweet potato, then grate them and place into a mixing bowl. Crack 1 egg into the mixing bowl, add a pinch of salt and pepper and mix well. Heat up the olive oil in a frying pan over a medium heat. Cup half the rosti mixture in your hand and make into a mini flat disc, gently squeeze out some of the liquid and place into the frying pan. Repeat the same process for the other rosti. Cook for 2-3 minutes per side, or until they are golden brown on both sides. Meanwhile, add a pinch of salt and a tsp of vinegar to boiling water. Create a swirl in the water and then quickly crack the second egg and add it to the water. Cook the egg for 90 to 120 secs, then remove from the water. Plate up the rosti and smoked salmon. Place the egg on top of the rosti. Sprinkle a little pepper over the salmon with a squeeze of lemon to finish.

DIETICIAN'S NOTES

A great balance of heart healthy fats, protein and vegetables - a great brunch meal that .will score you two of your

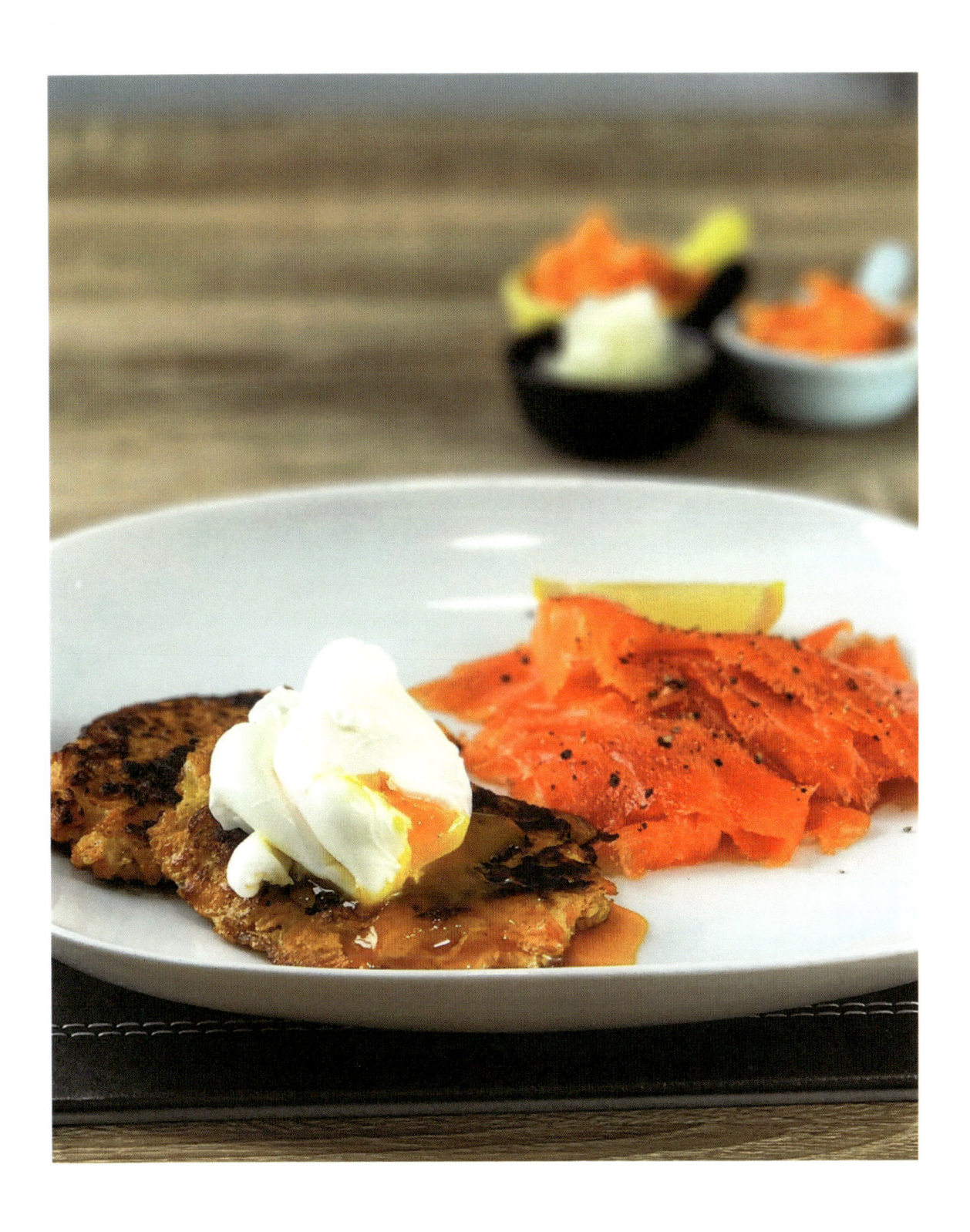

DARK CHOCOLATE OVERNIGHT OATS

(Per Serving) Calories 384 / Carbs 42g / Protein 36g / Fat 8g

Get your morning off to a nutritious start by preparing these oats in advance .... with fresh berries and fibre filled oats they will give you the energy you need to power through your morning. Yes - you CAN eat chocolate for breakfast!

Serves 1
Prep Time 10 mins
Cook Time Chill overnight

INGREDIENTS

1 square 70% Dark Chocolate (melted in the microwave)
200g (7oz) Plain Low Fat Greek Yogurt
15g (1/2oz) Chocolate Whey Protein
(can work with other flavours)
35g (1 1/4oz) Porridge Oats
30g (1oz) Blueberries
70g (2 1/2oz) Strawberries

HOW TO COOK IT

Melt the dark chocolate in a glass bowl over boiling water.

When melted, drizzle the dark chocolate around the inside of your chosen container.

Mix your Greek yogurt and protein powder together, then place half the mixture in the bottom of the container.

Add the oats to the container along with half the blueberries and chopped strawberries.

Finally, add the remainder of the Greek yogurt and protein powder mixture and top with the remaining fruit.

Seal the container and place in the fridge overnight to allow the oats to soften.

DIETICIAN'S NOTES

Oats are rich in beta glucan, a type of fibre that helps to regulate cholesterol levels. The mix of protein, carbohydrates and fibre in this breakfast should keep you energised throughout the morning.

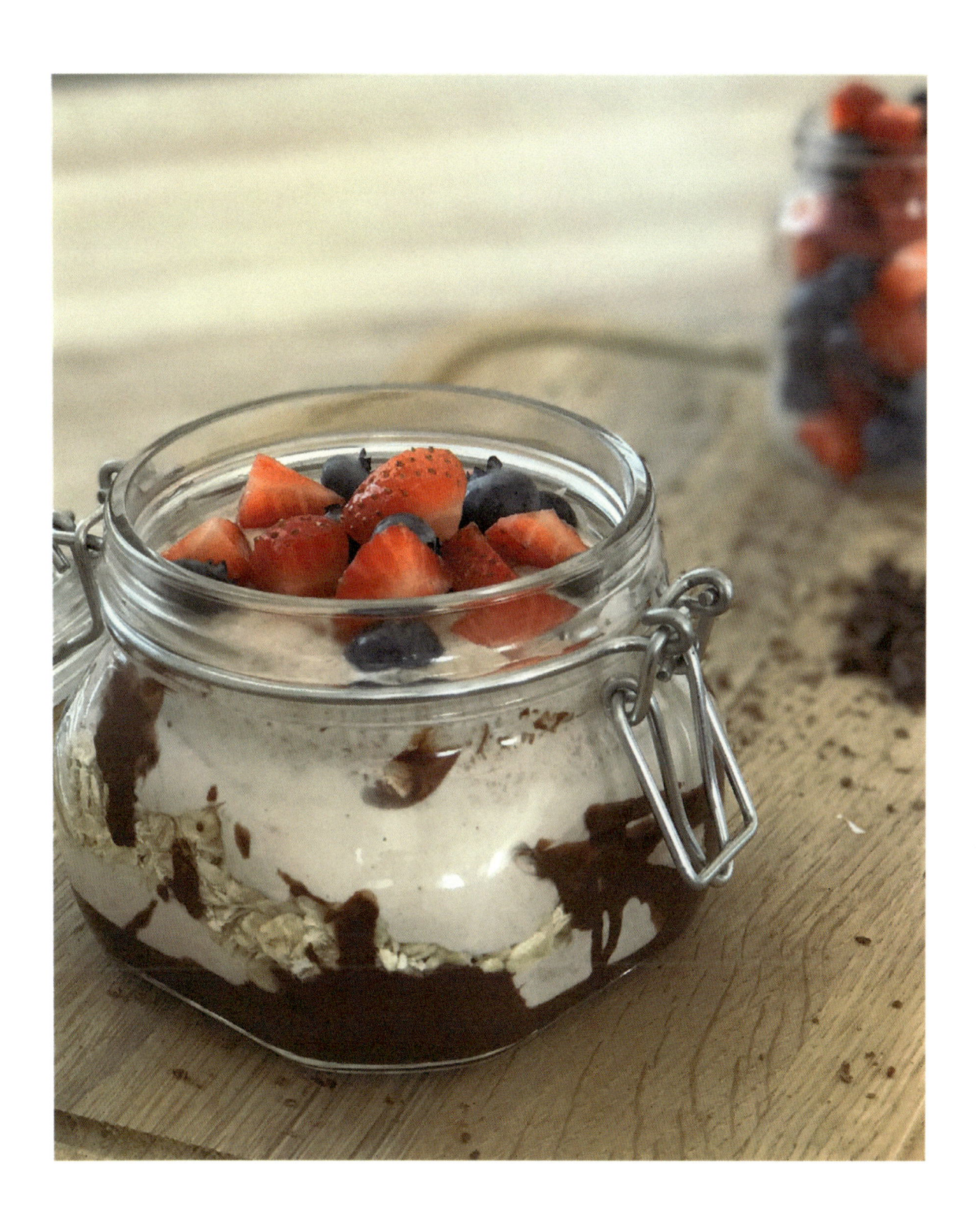

TOMATO EGG NESTS

(Per Serving) Calories 449 / Carbs 18g / Protein 47g / Fat 21g

Similar to the Mexican dish - huevos rancheros, this spicy tomato stew with eggs is the breakfast of champions! This recipe adds turkey rashers for even more protein. It's hearty, quick to make and a real crowd pleaser!

Serves 2
Prep Time 15 mins Cook Time 25 mins

INGREDIENTS

1 tsp Olive Oil
3 Turkey Rashers (cook and then cut into small pieces)
½ Large Onion (finely chopped)
1 Garlic Clove (finely chopped)
150g (5 1/4oz) Can of Tinned Tomatoes
1 tsp Tomato Purée
¼ tsp Cumin Powder
½ tsp Red Chilli Flakes
½ tsp Coriander (cilantro) Powder
Pinch Salt (to taste)
Pinch of Black Pepper (to taste)
2 Large Eggs
20g (3/4oz) Feta Cheese (roughly chopped)
Fresh Coriander (cilantro) (for garnishing)

HOW TO COOK IT

Heat half of the olive oil in a pan over a medium heat and cook the turkey rashers for 2-3 minutes per side. Then remove from the heat and chop into small pieces.

Heat the remainder of the olive oil in the pan. Chop up the onion and add to the pan.

Peel and finely chop the garlic. When the onion starts to brown, add the garlic and cook for 1 minute.

Then add the tinned tomatoes and tomato purée. Cook for another 1 minute.

Add in the turkey rashers, cumin, red chilli flakes, coriander (cilantro) powder, salt and pepper and stir.

Create holes in the mixture and crack the eggs into those holes.

Sprinkle with chopped up feta cheese and cook for 2 minutes.

Place the pan under the grill for 4-5 minutes to finish. Make sure eggs are cooked.

Sprinkle the fresh coriander (cilantro) over the top and serve

DIETICIAN'S NOTES

A low carbohydrates, protein rich breakfast rich in antioxidants, which help your body's immune defences. Add a side of toast if you're pre or post workout.

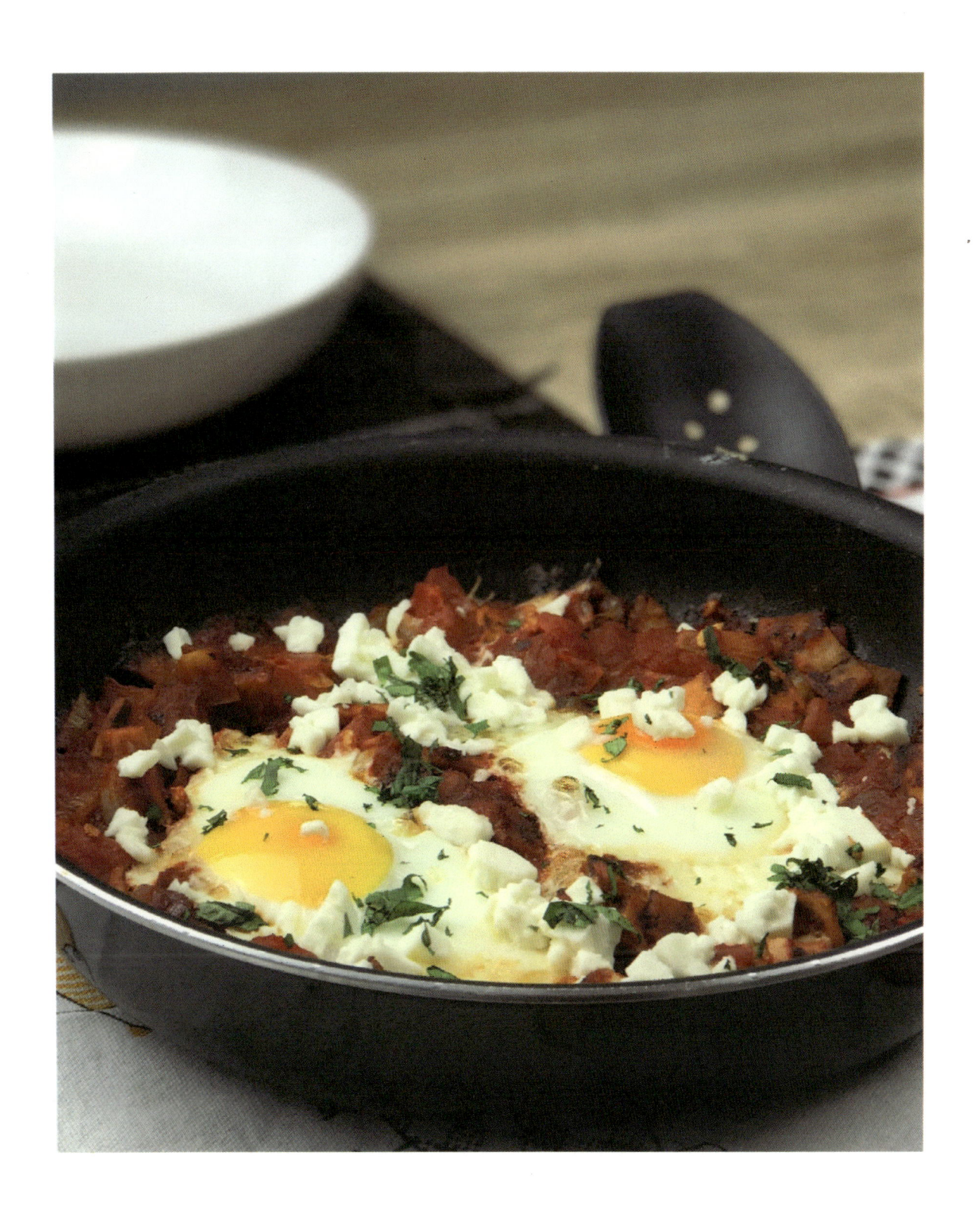

BREAKFAST SMOOTHIE

(Per Serving) Calories 480 / Carbs 35g / Protein 40g / Fat 20g

You wouldn't think that berries would go well with greens, like avocado and spinach, but they do! This delicious smoothie is packed with antioxidant berries as well as oats, peanut butter, banana and protein powder. You'll easily get to lunchtime without snacking!

Serves 1 Prep Time 5 mins Cook Time 1 mins **INGREDIENTS** 20g (3/4oz) Raspberries 20g (3/4oz) Blueberries 20g (3/4oz) Strawberries 30g (1oz) Spinach 30g (1oz) Oats 40g (1 1/2oz) Protein Powder 15g (1/2oz) Peanut Butter 1/3 Banana ¼ Avocado 1/2 Pint Water	**HOW TO COOK IT** Add the raspberries, blueberries, strawberries, spinach, oats, protein powder and peanut butter to the blender. Peel the banana, remove the avocado from its skin (removing the stone) before putting them both in the blender, along with the water. Blend until smooth. Note: Use frozen fruit for a colder more smoothie-like drink. Plus, they don't go off if they are frozen!

DIETICIAN'S NOTES

This fruit and vegetables packed smoothie provides two of your five-a-day. Adding protein powder means you'll stay fuller longer. A great grab and go choice.

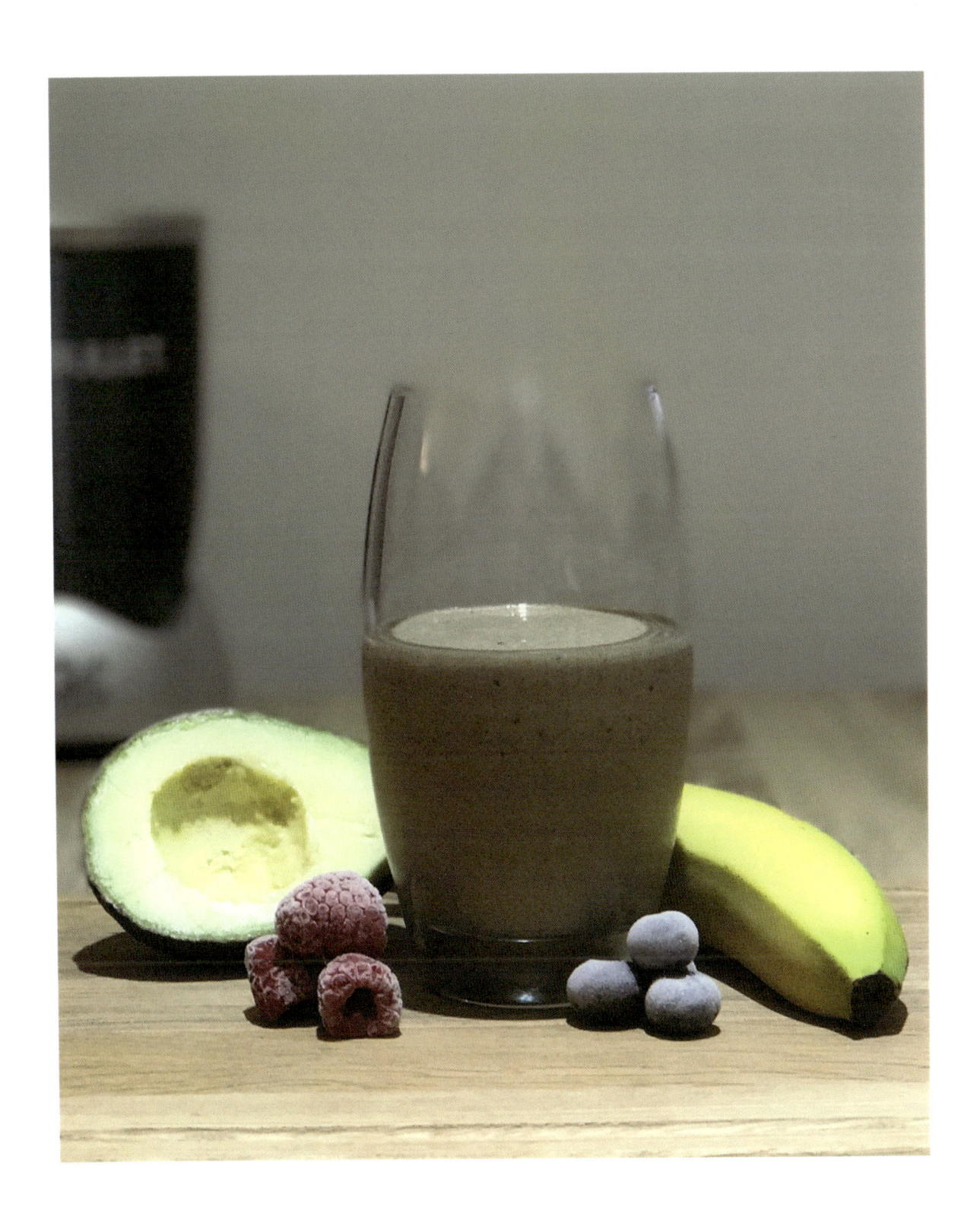

AVOCADO, BACON & EGG ON TOAST

(Per Serving) Calories 386 / Carbs 17g / Protein 30g / Fat 22g

Just like Eggs Benedict, but without the high-calorie Hollandaise! Runny poached eggs, crispy bacon and avocado are the perfect breakfast/lunch combination. Start your day in the right way with this simple yet superior dish!

Serves 2 Prep Time 5 mins Cook Time 10 mins **INGREDIENTS** 4 Smoked Bacon Medallions 2 Wholegrain Seeded Bread Slices Pinch of Salt 1 tsp Vinegar 4 Medium Eggs 1 Avocado	**HOW TO COOK IT** Put a saucepan of water on the heat and bring to the boil. Put the bacon under the grill and cook for 4 minutes per side or until done. Place the bread in the toaster and toast. Add a pinch of salt and a tsp of vinegar to the boiling water. Create a swirl in the water and then quickly crack the eggs into the water. Cook the eggs for 90 to 120 secs then remove from the water. Halve the avocado, remove the stone and mash both halves of the avocado. Spread the whole avocado between both slices of toast. Place the cooked bacon on top of the avocado. Place the cooked eggs on top of the bacon and serve.

DIETICIAN'S NOTES

Research has found that eating two eggs for breakfast can lower levels of hunger hormones more effectively than a breakfast of oatmeal. Switch bacon for salmon to benefit from anti-inflammatory omega-3.

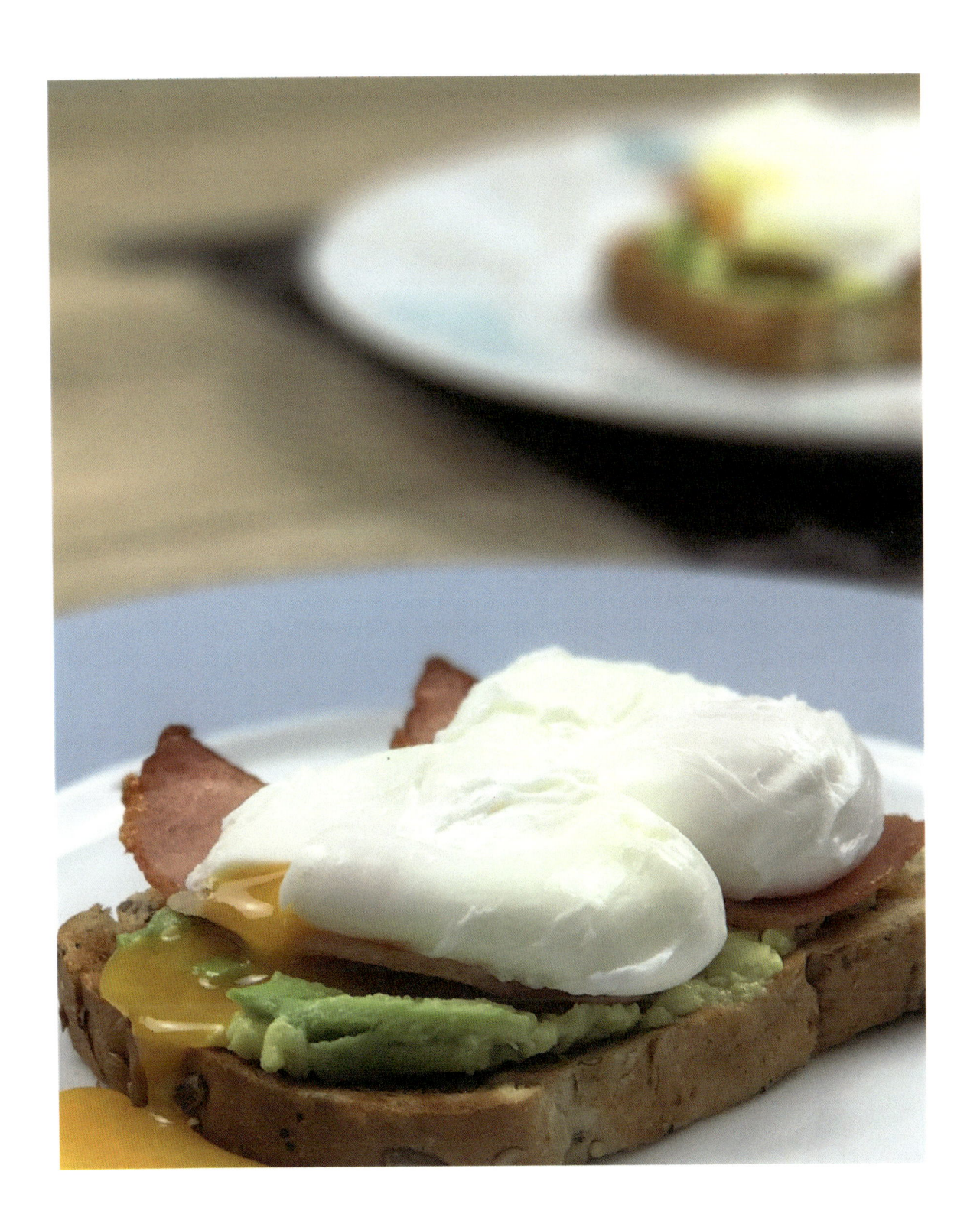

CHICKEN & SWEET POTATO HASH

(Per Serving) Calories 361 / Carbs 31g / Protein 39g / Fat 9g

This hash is a real treat for the taste buds, it's also super quick and easy to make in only twenty minutes. The sweet potato, apple and cinnamon go really well with the chicken, which is served with more vegetables. Add a poached egg on top for extra protein!

Serves 2 Prep Time 5 mins Cook Time 15 mins ## INGREDIENTS 310g (11oz) Chicken 1 tbsp Olive Oil 200g (7oz) Sweet Potato 1 Cox Apple 2 tsp Cinnamon Pinch of Salt (to taste) Pinch of Pepper (to taste) 10 tbsp of Water 50g (1 3/4oz) Asparagus 50g (1 3/4oz) Baby corn	## HOW TO COOK IT Cut the chicken into medium chunks. Heat the olive oil over a medium heat. Add the chicken to the pan for 2-3 minutes, searing all sides of the chicken. Peel and chop up the sweet potato into 1 cm chunks and the apple into slightly bigger chunks. Add them both to pan along with the cinnamon and salt and pepper (to taste). Cook for 12-15 minutes or until the chicken is cooked and the potato is slightly soft. Use the water, 1 tbsp at a time, to keep a little bit of liquid in the pan to soften the apple and potato. Cook your asparagus and baby corn (or preferred vegetables) and then serve.

DIETICIAN'S NOTES

Teaming fibre rich carbohydrates, like sweet potato with protein rich foods is a smart way to maintain steady energy levels. Score top marks by adding extra vegetables.

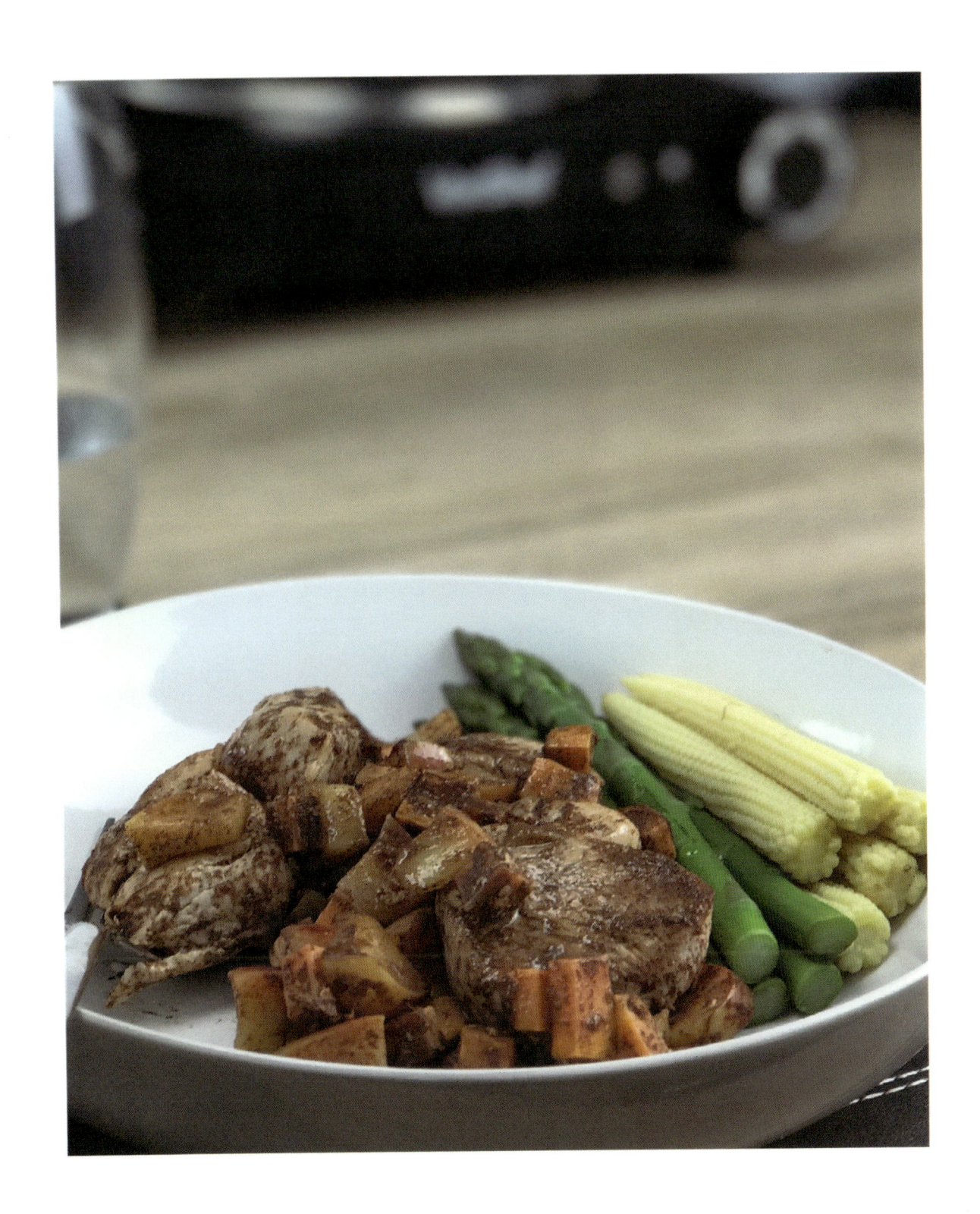

CHICKEN, PARMA HAM, AVOCADO & FETA SALAD

(Per Serving) Calories 418 / Carbs 3g / Protein 52g / Fat 22g

There are so many delicious flavours and textures in this hearty salad - the buttery avocado and the crumbly feta complement the tender chicken and the salty parma ham perfectly. It's ideal for lunch or a light dinner.

Serves 1
Prep Time 5 mins Cook Time 10 mins

INGREDIENTS

1 tsp Extra Virgin Olive Oil

160g (5 1/2oz) Chicken

20g (3/4oz) Feta Cheese

½ Avocado

2 Slices Parma Ham

2 Handfuls Salad Leaves

Pinch Salt & Pepper

1 tsp Balsamic Vinegar

HOW TO COOK IT

Heat ½ the olive oil in a frying on a medium heat.

Cut the chicken into small chunks and place in the pan. Cook for 4 minutes per side or until the chicken is cooked through.

Whilst the chicken is cooking, make the salad by chopping up the feta cheese, chopping up the avocado (after removing the skin and the stone) and roughly pulling apart the Parma Ham. Place these on top of your chosen salad leaves.

When the chicken is cooked, add it to the salad mixture, sprinkle with salt and pepper, add in the other half of the olive oil and the teaspoon of balsamic vinegar and mix well before serving.

DIETICIAN'S NOTES

A low carbohydrate lunch which should keep you feeling satisfied thanks to the high protein content. Throw in a handful of cherry tomatoes or roasted peppers to score an extra serving of vegetables.

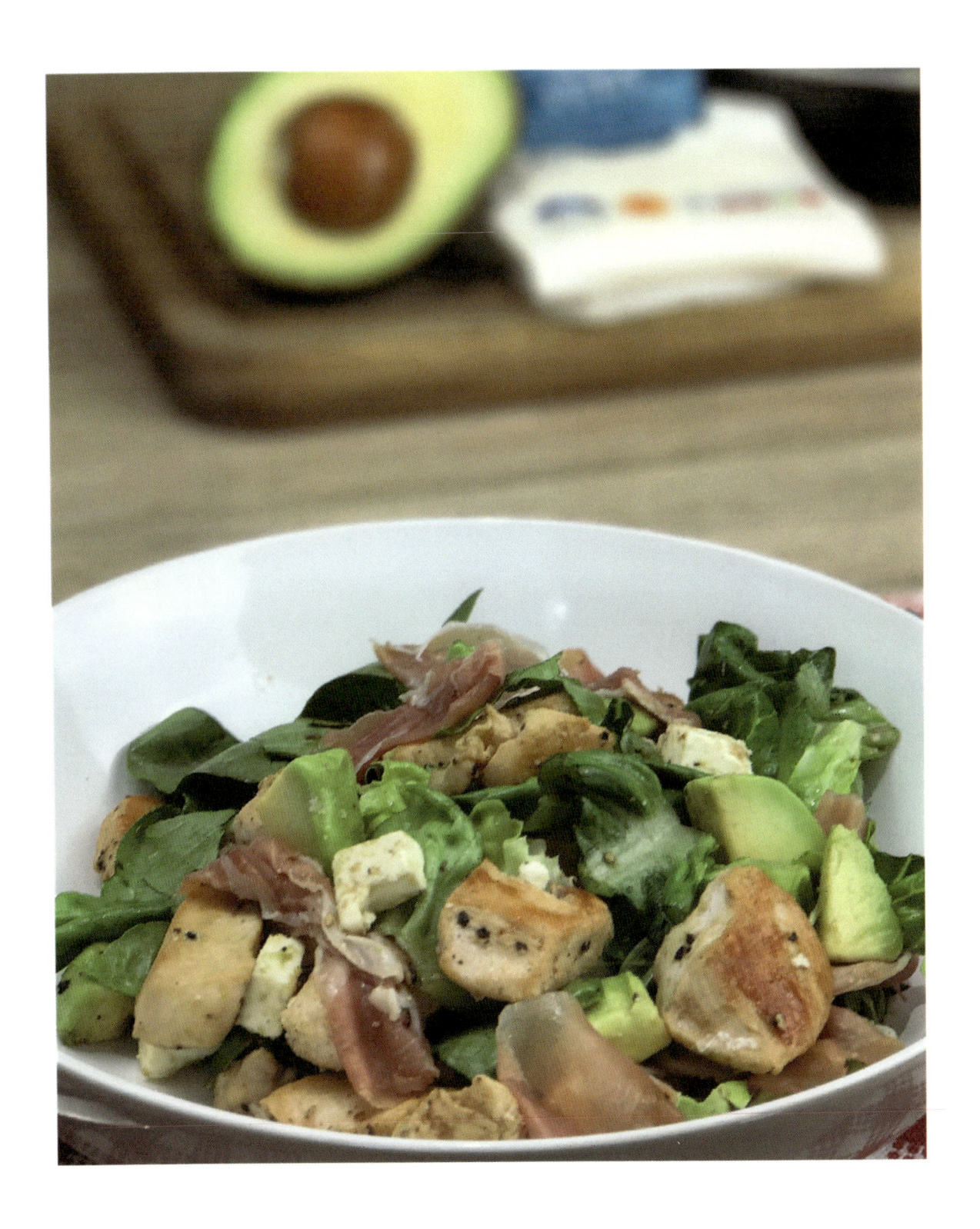

STUFFED PEPPERS

(Per Serving) Calories 289 / Carbs 22g / Protein 39g / Fat 5g

A quick and easy-to-make meal that won't leave you feeling stuffed! These protein-packed peppers combine lean turkey mince, brown rice and fresh vegetables for the perfect healthy weeknight meal. Packed with antioxidants and vitamin C rich bell peppers to support immune function

Serves 1 Prep Time 15 mins Cook Time 25 mins ## INGREDIENTS 40g (1 1/2oz) Brown Rice (14g or 1/2oz dry weight) 2 Bell Peppers 1 tsp Olive Oil ½ Onion 1 Garlic Clove 135g (4 3/4oz) Turkey Mince 175g (6 1/4oz) Tinned Chopped Tomatoes 1/2 tsp Mixed Herbs Pinch of Salt (to taste) Pinch of Pepper (to taste)	## HOW TO COOK IT Preheat oven to 200°C (392°F). Cook the rice as per instructions on the packet. To save time, use microwave rice) Chop off the top of the peppers and remove all the seeds from inside. Heat up the olive oil in a frying pan over a medium heat. Chop up the onion and cook for 2 minutes, then finely chop the garlic and cook for 30 seconds. Add the turkey mince and cook for 4-5 minutes. Add the pre-cooked rice, tinned tomatoes, mixed herbs, salt and pepper, then cook for a further 4 minutes. Add the mixture to the peppers and place in the preheated oven for 25 minutes. Leave to stand for 3 minutes before serving.

DIETICIAN'S NOTES

A tasty meal which ticks off three of your five-a-day. Canned tomatoes are a rich source of a potent antioxidant called lycopene – adding a splash of olive oil helps your body absorb this nutrient.

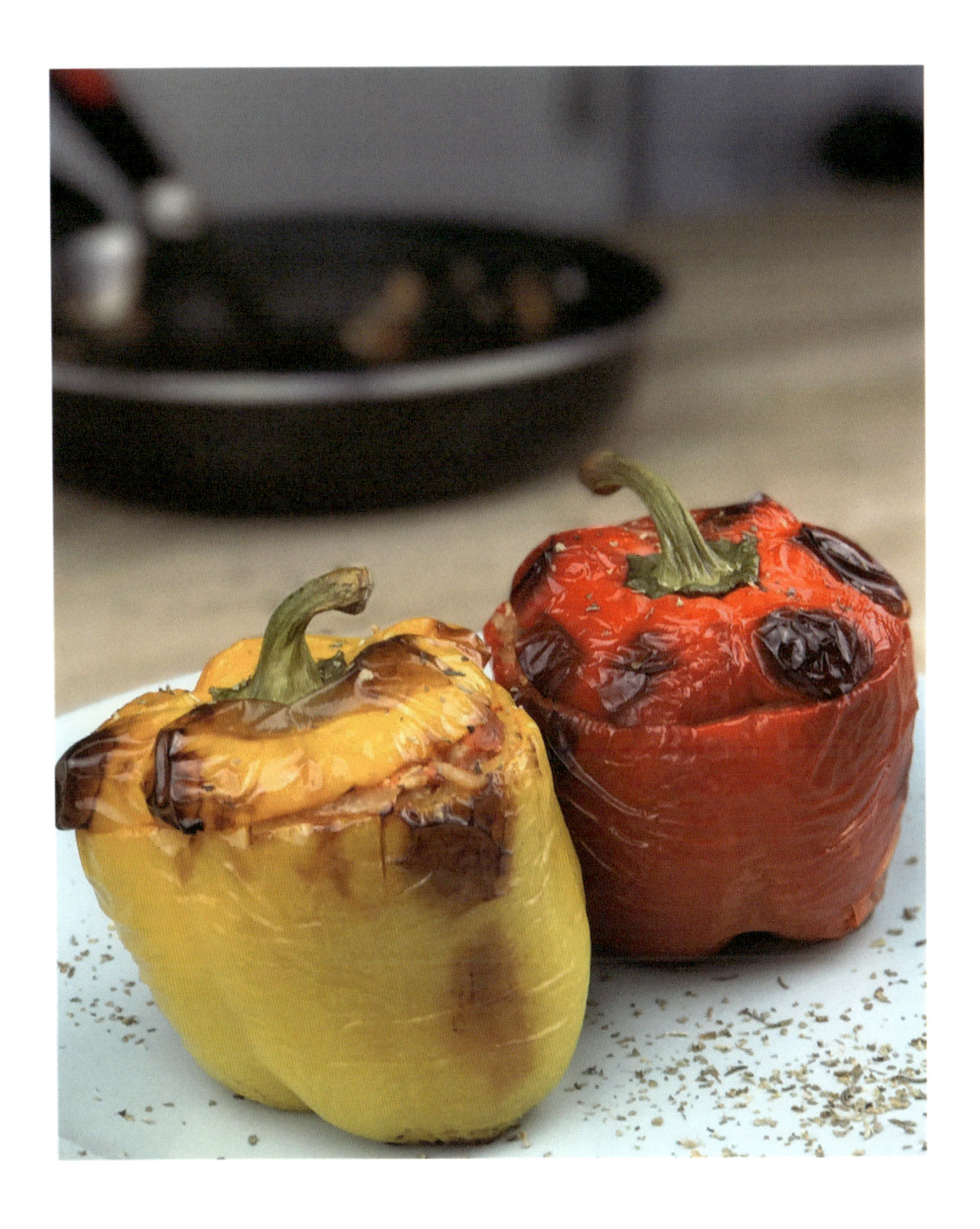

ORANGE & OREGANO CHICKEN SALAD

(Per Serving) Calories 391 / Carbs 16g / Protein 39g / Fat 19g

Chicken generally goes well with citrus flavours and works really well with orange! This healthy and filling salad contains two of your five-a-day and looks like a rainbow on a plate, which is a sign of an antioxidant rich meal.

Serves 2
Prep Time 10 mins Cook Time 10 mins

INGREDIENTS

2 Large Oranges (juiced)
1 tbsp Soy Sauce
300g (10 1/2oz) Chicken Breast
100g (3 1/2oz) Broccoli
1 Carrot
100g (3 1/2oz) Radishes
½ Red Onion
100g (3 1/2oz) Red Peppers
100g (3 1/2oz) Cucumber
1 tbsp Olive Oil
Zest of ½ an Orange
1 tbsp Apple Cider Vinegar
1 tsp Dried Oregano
25g (3/4oz) Pine Nuts

HOW TO COOK IT

For the marinade: Add the juice from 1 orange and the soy sauce to a mixing bowl.

Halve the chicken breasts, add to the marinade and put to one side.

Halve or quarter the broccoli (depending on the size) and add to boiling water for 3 minutes, then run under cold water to cool.

Add these ingredients to a mixing bowl: broccoli, peeled and grated carrot, grated radishes, peeled & grated onion, sliced pepper, peeled & sliced cucumber and put to one side.

Add a teaspoon of olive oil to a frying pan over a medium heat. Cook the chicken for 4 minutes per side or until cooked through.

Make the salad dressing by adding these ingredients together: orange zest, 3 tablespoons of orange juice, apple cider vinegar, ½ tablespoon of olive oil and dried oregano.

Plate up your salad, add ½ the pine nuts to each dish, add the chicken and then pour over your salad dressing.

DIETICIAN'S NOTES

Citrus fruits, carrots and green vegetables are top protectors against heart disease. Adding pine nuts to this dish is a great way to add healthy fats.

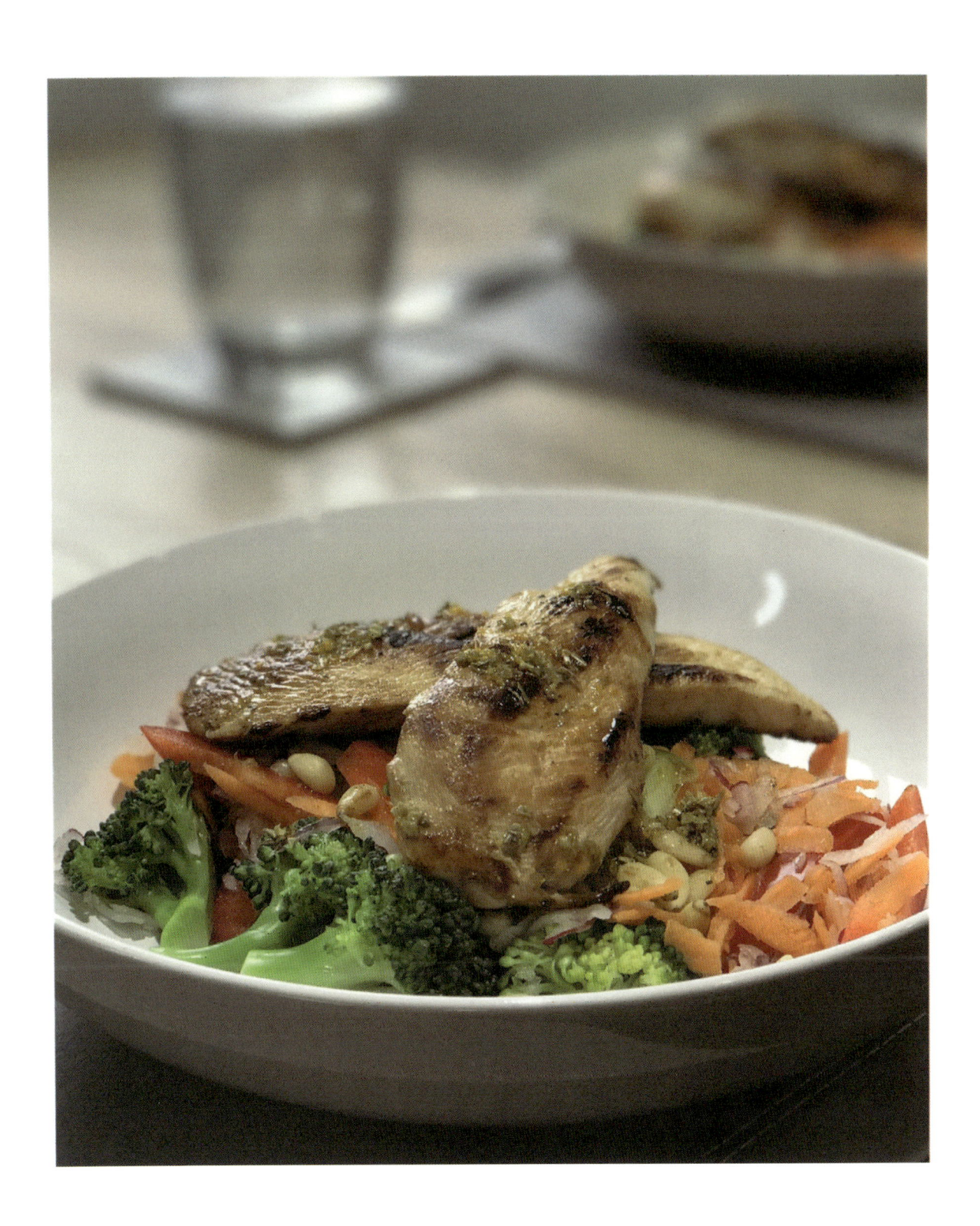

CHINESE SPICED DUCK SALAD

(Per Serving) Calories 329 / Carbs 9g / Protein 35g / Fat 17g

This exotic duck salad has got it all going on - juicy fruit, spice, crunch and delicious crispy duck. It's quick to make and packed full of flavour. A tasty, filling lunch or dinner that will put the brakes on hunger.

Serves 2 Prep Time 10 mins Cook Time 10 mins **INGREDIENTS** 2 Large Duck Breasts 1 tbsp Chinese Five Spice Powder ½ Ripe Mango 2 Spring Onions (scallions) 1 Sprig Fresh Coriander (cilantro) 2 tbsp Pomegranates A Few Sprigs Watercress 1 Little Gem Lettuce ½ Lime (Juiced) 2 tsp Sesame Oil	**HOW TO COOK IT** Score the skin of both duck breasts and then sprinkle the tablespoon of Chinese five spice on the duck breasts and rub in. Place in a pan on a medium heat, skin side down first. Cook for 3 minutes per side then remove from the heat and slice the duck into centimetre slices. Pour away the fat from the pan and then wipe it clean with a paper towel. Return the sliced duck to the pan and cook for 2 minutes. Meanwhile, peel and slice the mango into cubes. Trim and slice the spring onions (scallions). Chop the coriander (cilantro) Place the 3 ingredients above in a mixing bowl along with the pomegranates, watercress and the sliced duck and mix it all together. Place the little gem salad into bowls for serving. Divide the duck mixture into the two bowls, squeeze the lime and drizzle the sesame oil over each dish and serve.

DIETICIAN'S NOTES

Duck is rich in iron, which helps fight fatigue. Aim to keep red meat intake to ~ 500 grams cooked weight per week - this leaves plenty of room for fish and plant-based meals

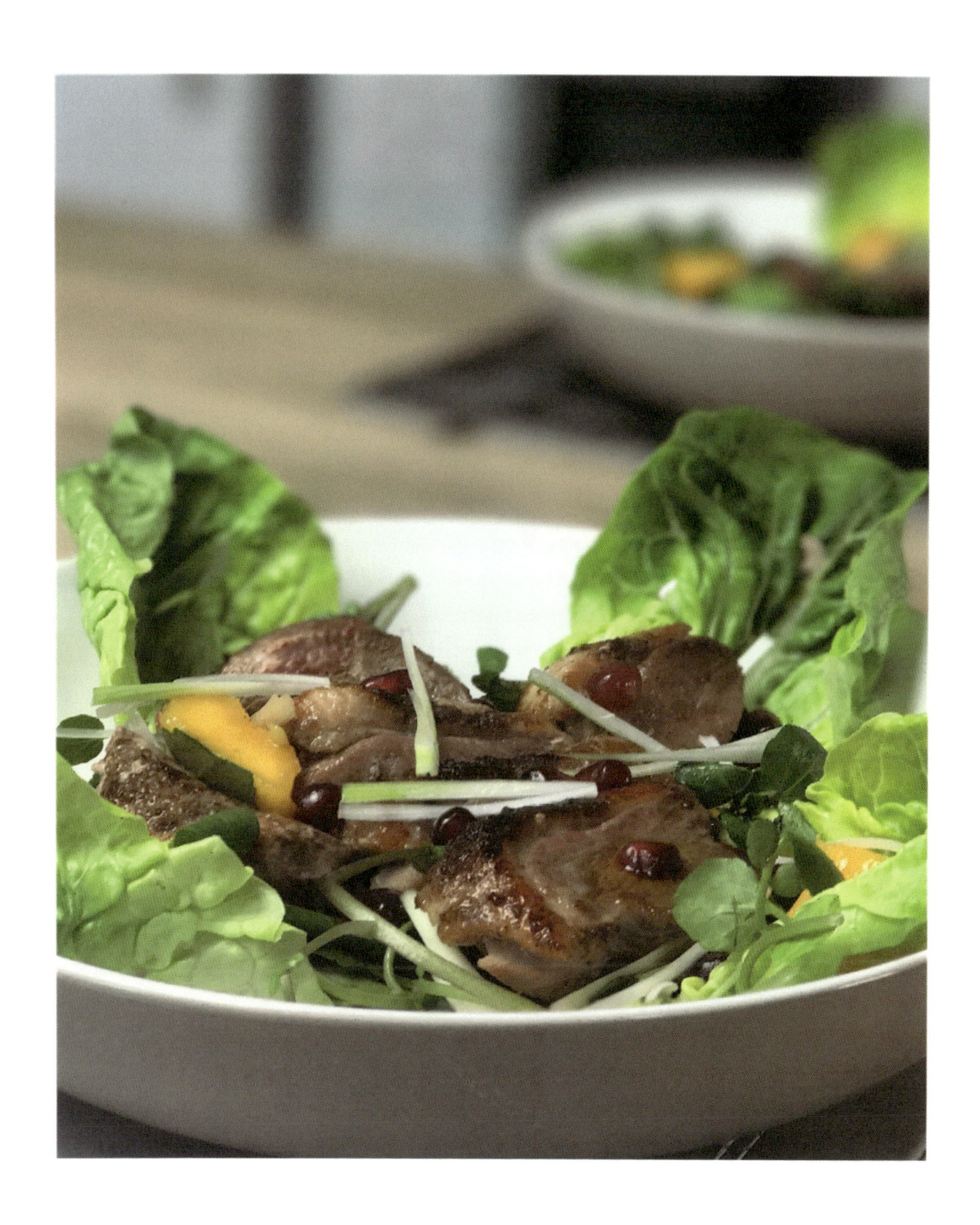

CHILLI CHICKEN AND AVOCADO WRAP

(Per Serving) Calories 558 / Carbs 32g / Protein 40g / Fat 30g

If you love fajitas, you'll love this lunchtime wrap. Pan-fry lean chicken breast with lime, chilli and garlic, then pile on top of mashed avocado on a wholemeal wrap. The avocado cools the chilli and creates a delicious combination!

Serves 2 Prep Time 10 mins Cook Time 10 mins **INGREDIENTS** 1 Garlic Clove ½ tsp Chilli Powder ½ Lime (Juice) 300g (10 1/2oz) Chicken Breast 1 tsp Olive Oil 1 Avocado 2 Wholemeal Wraps 40g (1 1/2oz) Roasted Peppers Coriander (cilantro)	**HOW TO COOK IT** Finely chop the garlic and place in a mixing bowl along with the chilli powder and the juice from ½ a lime. Cut the chicken into pieces and add to the mixing bowl. Cover the chicken with the marinade and put to one side (marinade for longer if you want a stronger flavour). Heat the olive oil in a pan over a medium heat before adding the chicken. Cook the chicken for 5 minutes per side or until cooked through. Halve the avocado and remove the stone. Mash both halves up with a fork and then spread evenly between 2 wraps. Lay the cooked chicken on top of the avocado, followed by the roasted peppers. Sprinkle over some coriander (cilantro) and wrap them up, cut in half and serve.

DIETICIAN'S NOTES

Choosing wholegrains (like these wraps) is a great choice when it comes to starchy foods - the fibre they contain helps regulate cholesterol and can protect against the risk of bowel cancer.

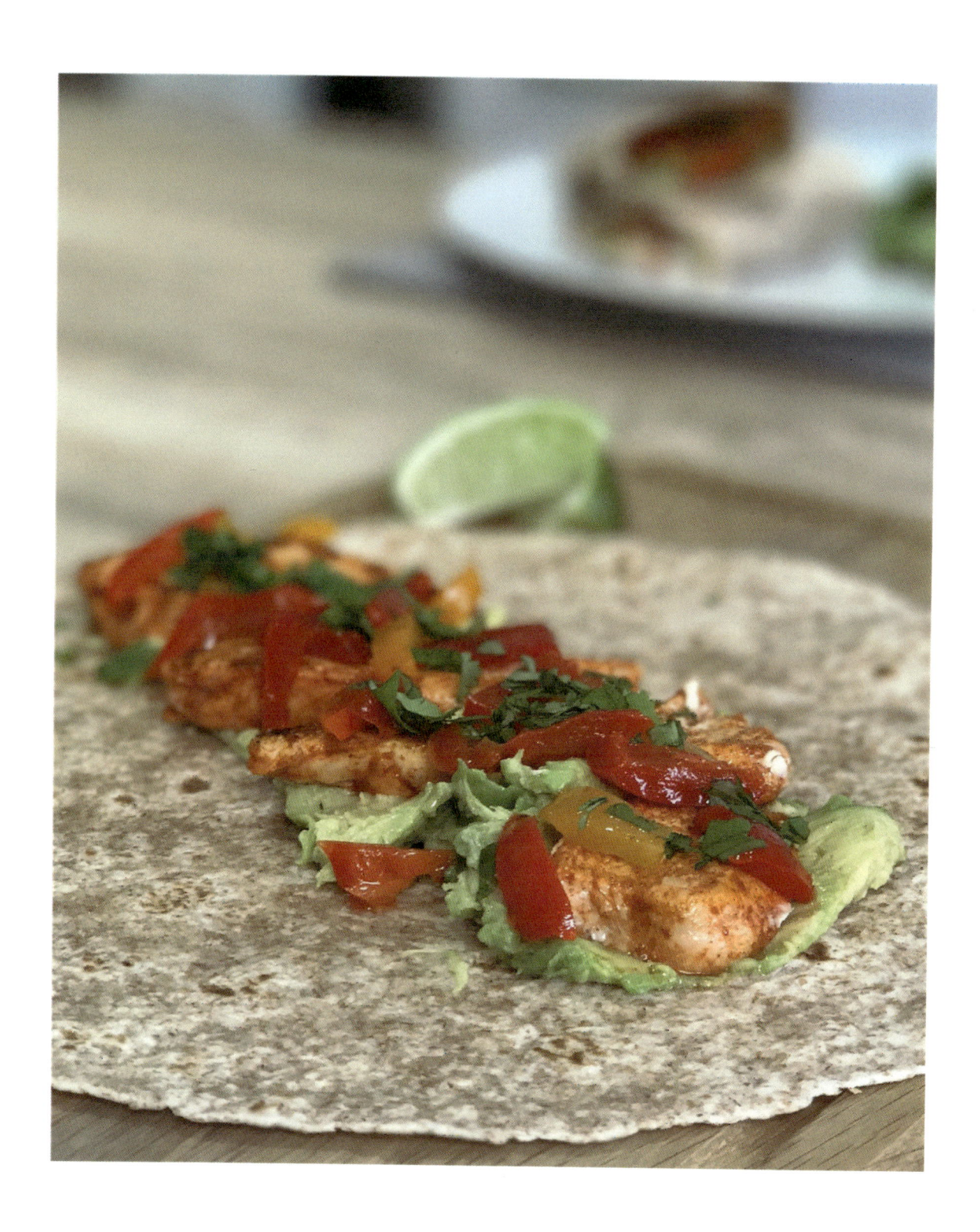

GINGER & SPRING ONION STEAMED COD

(Per Serving) Calories 319 / Carbs 35g / Protein 38g / Fat 3g

An Asian inspired approach to cooking fish - steam cod with pak choi, ginger, garlic and rice wine and serve topped with crunchy spring onions and fragrant coriander, basmati rice and broccoli. The flavours are light and zingy - a tasty and different way to eat cod!

Serves 2 Prep Time 10 mins Cook Time 20 mins ## INGREDIENTS 6 Leaves of Pak Choi 360g (12 3/4oz) Cod Fillet 1 Large Garlic Clove 5cm Thinly Sliced Ginger (peeled) 2 tsp Light Soy Sauce 1 ½ tsp Mirin Rice Wine 100g (3 1/2oz) Broccoli 250g (8 3/4oz) Cooked Basmati Rice 1 Spring Onion (scallion) Pinch of Coriander (cilantro) ½ a Lime	## HOW TO COOK IT Preheat oven to 200°C (392°F). Tear off 2 pieces of foil and lay on a flat surface. Lay your Pak Choi into the centre of your foil. Place your cod on top of the Pak Choi. Finely chop the garlic and ginger and place on top of the cod. Drizzle over the soy sauce and Mirin rice wine. Create a parcel out of the foil, make sure the foil is secure at the top and sides. Place in the preheated oven for 20 minutes. Cook the broccoli for 5 minutes. Cook the rice as per the instructions on the packet. Plate up the food, add chopped spring onion (scallion) and coriander (cilantro) to the cod along with a squeeze of lime. Finish off by pouring the juice from the foil over the fish and serve.

DIETICIAN'S NOTES

Cod is a good source of vitamin 12, which we need for making healthy red blood cells. White fish is also rich in protein but low in fat, making this a low calorie but satisfying meal.

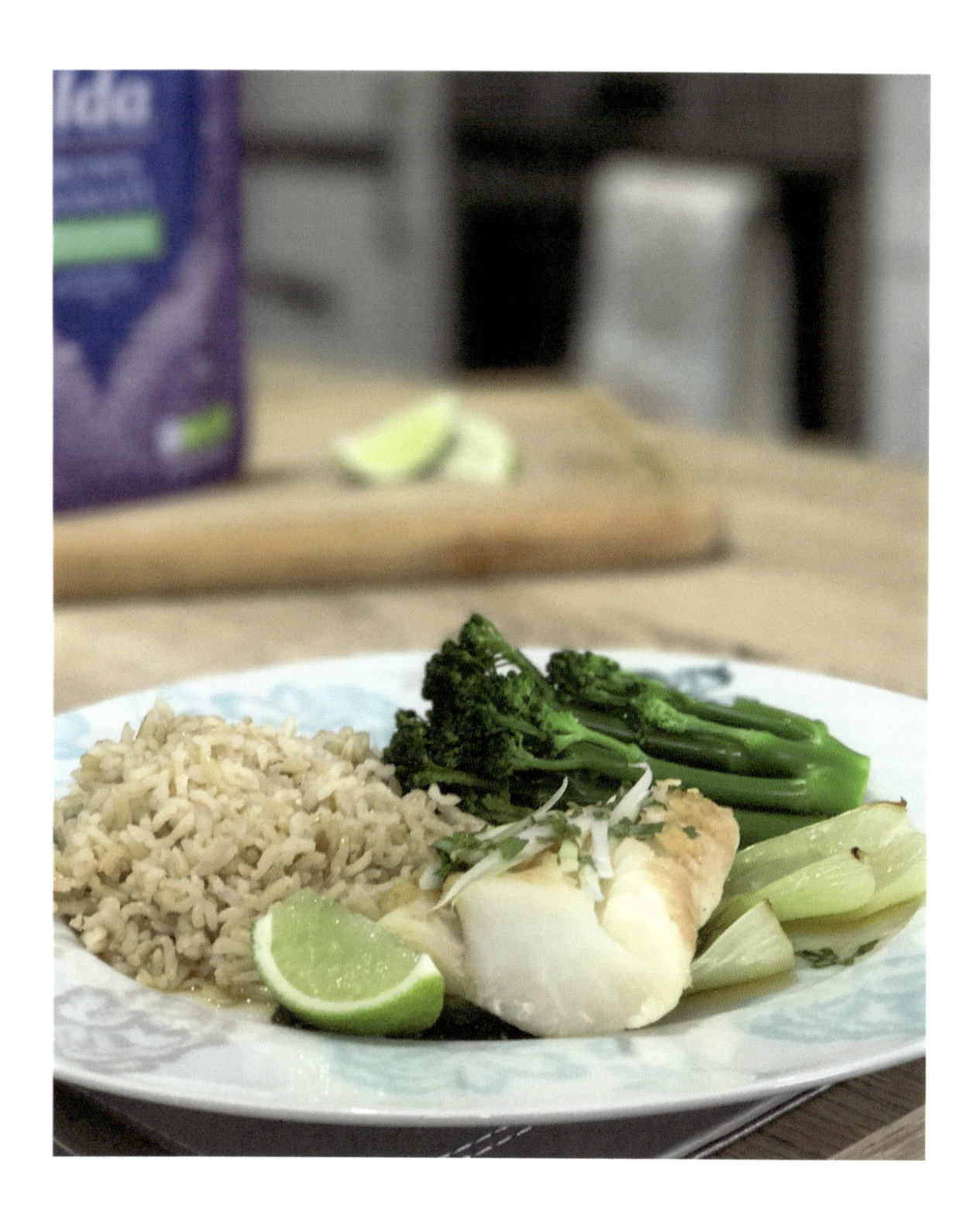

CHICKEN STIR FRY

(Per Serving) Calories 351 / Carbs 18g / Protein 45g / Fat 11g

Get that wok sizzling and enjoy throwing in ingredients to create this popular classic! The noodles give this dish a great protein punch. Ginger, garlic and soy sauce add the well-loved Asian flavours!

Serves 2
Prep Time 5 mins Cook Time 15 mins

INGREDIENTS

1 tsp Olive Oil
½ Onion
1 Clove Garlic
Ginger, thumb size
250g (8 3/4oz) Chicken
75g (2 1/2oz) Carrots
100g (3 1/2oz) Red Bell Pepper
100g (3 1/2oz) Sugar Snap Peas
100g (3 1/2oz) Tenderstem Broccoli
2 tbsp Light Soy Sauce
½ Chicken Stock Cube
100ml (1/2cup) Boiling Water
½ tsp Corn-starch
115g (4oz) Protein Noodles

HOW TO COOK IT

Heat the olive oil in a wok or frying pan on a medium heat.

Roughly chop the onion and add to the pan for 1 minute.

Peel and finely chop the garlic and ginger and add to the pan for 1 minute.

Cut the chicken into chunks, add to the pan and cook for 4 minutes or until the chicken starts to brown.

Grate the carrot, roughly chop up the pepper and add to the pan, cook for 1 minute before adding the sugar snaps and broccoli, then cook for a further 2 minutes. Now add the soy sauce and cook for another 2 minutes, until vegetables are crisp-tender.

Dissolve the ½ chicken stock in boiling water, then dissolve the cornstarch in the stock Add this to the pan (10tbsp = roughly 100ml) and simmer for 3 minutes, until sauce thickens.

1 minute from serving, add 1 pack (115g) protein noodles and mix in.

Serve the dish.

DIETICIAN'S NOTES

A vegetable packed stir-fry that ticks off 2 of your 5-a-day - a habit linked to a lower risk of heart disease & cancer. Add extra ginger to help muscle recovery; research shows it has anti-inflammatory

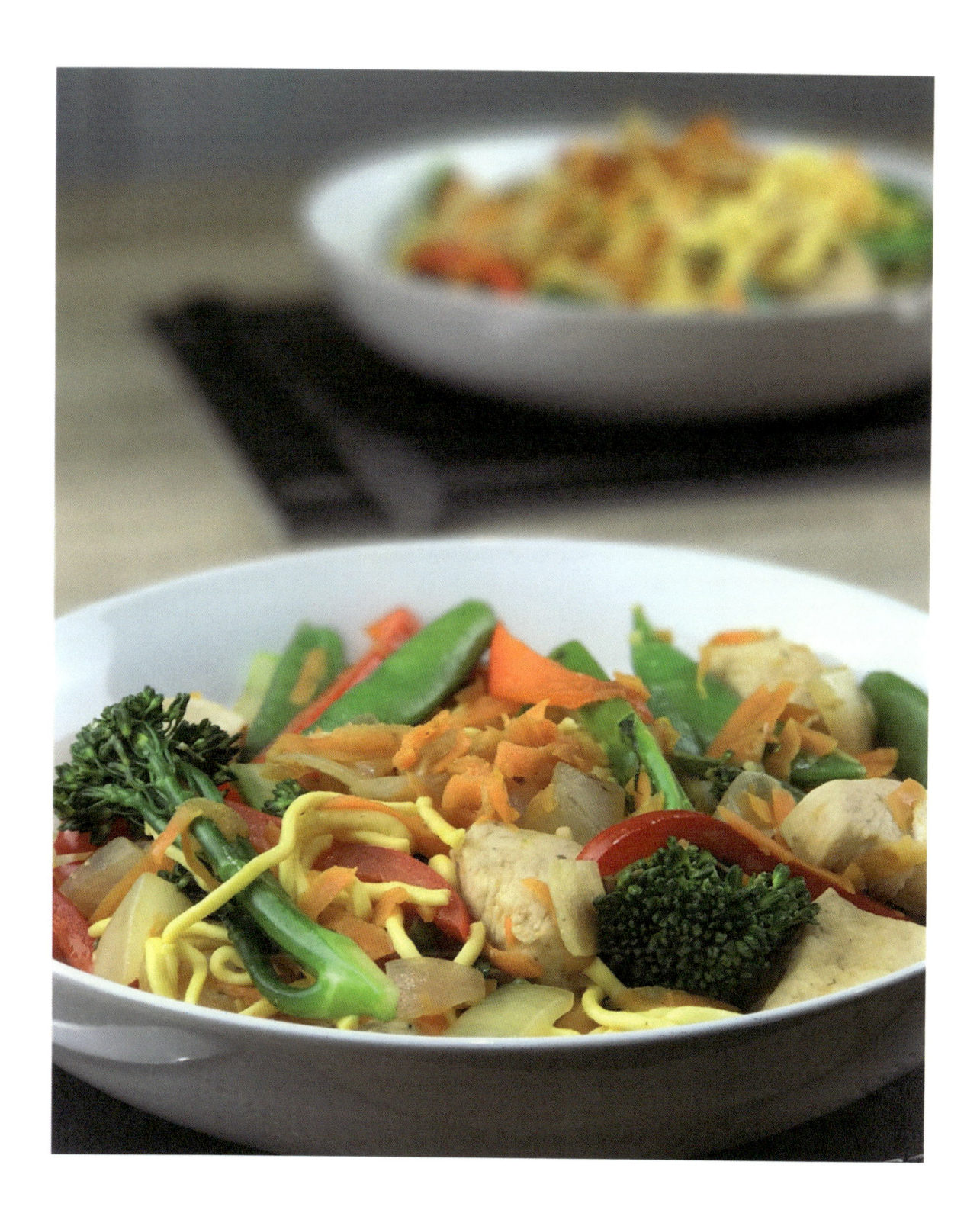

STEAK SALAD

(Per Serving) Calories 427 / Carbs 7g / Protein 39g / Fat 27g

Treat yourself with a juicy sirloin steak on a bed of crunchy salad! Crumbly feta cheese adds even more flavour into this tasty lunch or evening meal. A different way to enjoy salad that's perfect for the steak lover! The balsamic vinaigrette finishes it off perfectly.

Serves 2 Prep Time 5 mins Cook Time 10 mins **INGREDIENTS** 2tsp Olive Oil 320g (11 1/4oz) Sirloin Steak Salt & Pepper 100g (3 1/2oz) Red Onion 100g (3 1/2oz) Baby Cherry Tomatoes 100g (3 1/2oz) Cucumber 2tsp Apple Cider Vinegar 30g (1oz) Feta Cheese	**HOW TO COOK IT** Heat half the olive oil in a frying pan (medium heat). Season the steak with salt and pepper and cook to your liking in the pan, then leave to one side to rest. Meanwhile, peel and thinly slice the red onion. Run under water for one minute. Halve the tomatoes. Peel, halve and then slice the cucumber. Add the 3 ingredients to a mixing bowl along with the rest of the olive oil and apple cider vinegar then mix. Chop up the feta cheese and add to the salad mixture, then gently toss the salad before plating it up. Cut the steak and serve on the salad.

DIETICIAN'S NOTES

Steak is rich in iron, which is necessary for our bodies to make healthy red blood cells. If you're recovering from a workout, or want to add fibre to this dish, serve with a sweet potato.

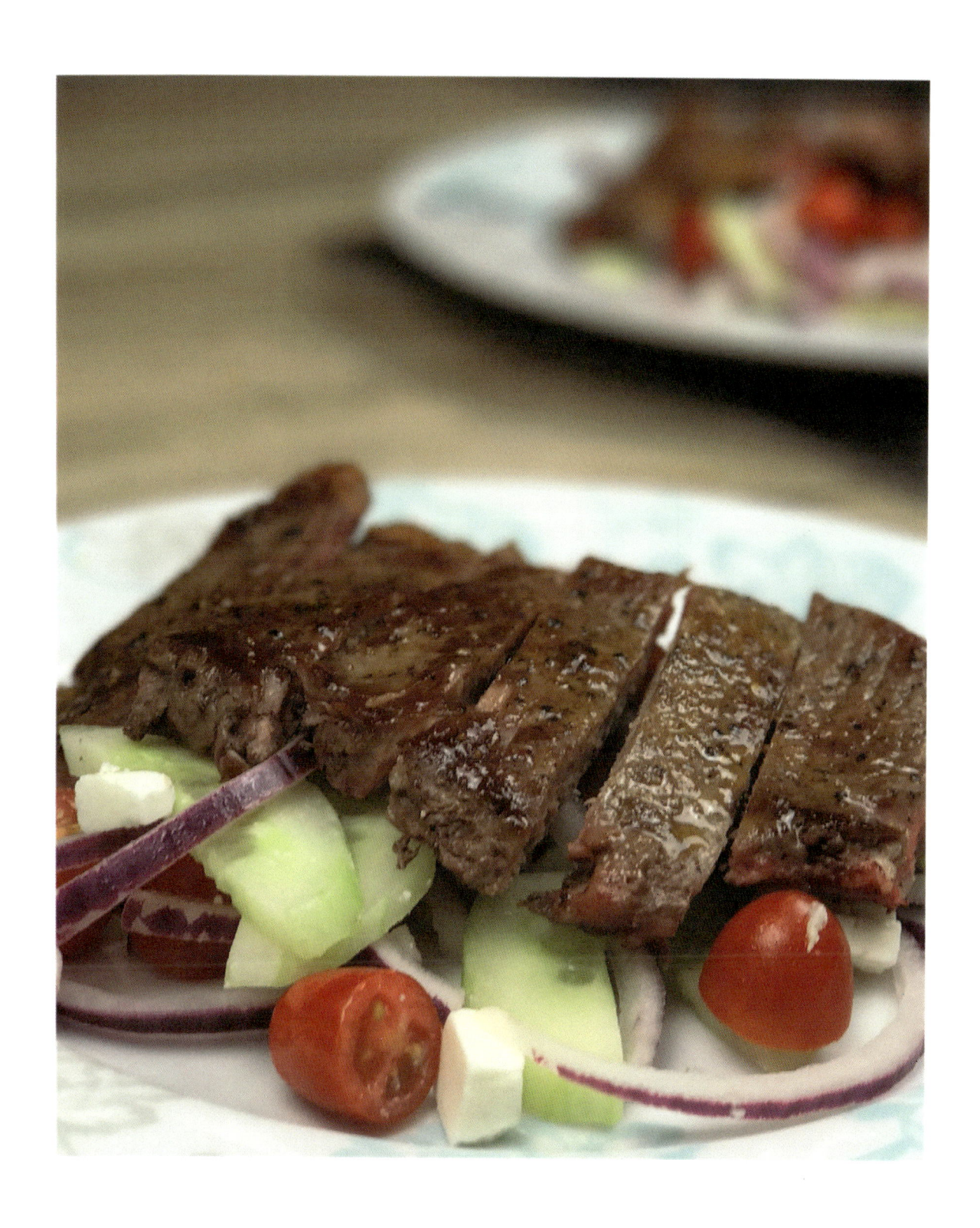

HASSELBACK FAJITA CHICKEN

(Per Serving) Calories 525 / Carbs 15g / Protein 60g / Fat 25g

If you're bored with the usual chicken dishes, this is definitely something different! Using a technique usually used for potatoes, Hasselback chicken is a low-carb way to enjoy Mexican flavours. It's a delicious and healthy weeknight dinner that takes no time to make!

Serves 2 Prep Time 10 mins Cook Time 20 mins ## INGREDIENTS 100g (3 1/2oz) Coloured Peppers 1 Red Onion 2 x 200g (7oz) Chicken Breasts 2 tsp Olive Oil 2 tsp Fajita Mix 50g (1 3/4oz) Cheddar Cheese 100g (3 1/2oz) Sweetcorn 100g (3 1/2oz) Broccoli 2 tbsp Soured Cream	## HOW TO COOK IT Thinly slice the peppers and onion. Make slits across the top of each chicken breast, approximately 1.5 cm apart. Cover each chicken breast with 1 tsp of olive oil and 1 tsp of fajita mix and rub in. Evenly place the pepper and onion slices into the slits you have created in the chicken. Place the chicken breasts onto a grill pan and grill on a medium heat for 15 mins. Grate the cheese and sprinkle onto of the chicken breasts and place back under the grill for 3 mins. Meanwhile, cook your vegetables. Plate up and spoon on your soured cream and tuck in.

DIETICIAN'S NOTES

Protein rich meals help us stay fuller longer, which can help with weight loss goals. Add extra vegetables for more fibre - a vital nutrient for the health of your digestive system.

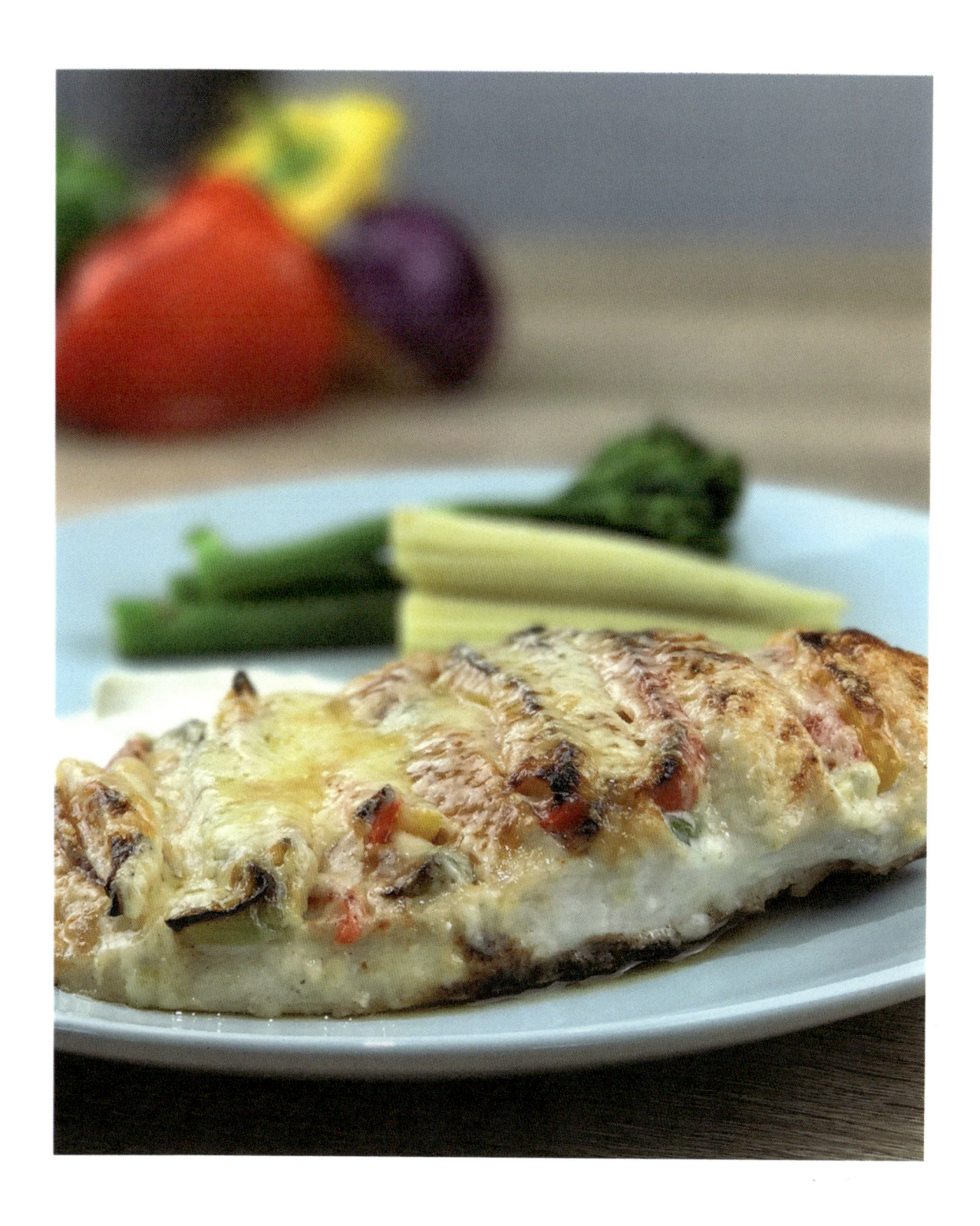

COD & ROASTED VEGETABLES

(Per Serving) Calories 480 / Carbs 37g / Protein 38g / Fat 20g

This one tray, healthy and simple fish dish will whisk you off to the Mediterranean with its flavours! The roasted vegetables are a great way to add flavour to white fish. Serve with asparagus and lemon for maximum flavour!

Serves 1 Prep Time 5 mins Cook Time 60 mins ## INGREDIENTS 150g (5 1/4oz) New Potatoes 50g (1 3/4oz) Carrots 50g (1 3/4oz) Peppers 50g (1 3/4oz) Shallots 1 ½ tbsp Olive Oil 1 tsp Paprika Salt & Pepper 2 Rosemary Stems 50g (1 3/4oz) Tomatoes 180g (6 1/4oz) Cod 2 Slices of Lemon 50g (1 3/4oz) Asparagus	## HOW TO COOK IT Preheat oven to 190°C. Halve the potatoes, peel and chop the carrots, cut the pepper into 3cm cubes, peel the shallots and add them all to a roasting tin. Add a tablespoon of olive oil, a teaspoon of paprika and a pinch of salt and pepper. Mix well, put the rosemary on top and place in the preheated oven for 20mins. Remove from the oven and mix, then place it back in the oven for a further 20mins. Remove once again from the oven and mix. Then add the tomatoes. Place the cod on top of the vegetables, cover with a teaspoon of olive oil, salt and pepper and sliced lemon before putting back into the oven for a final 20mins. Cook your asparagus for 3-4 minutes and plate up all the food.

DIETICIAN'S NOTES

Three of your five-a-day in one meal

-score! Olive oil contains high levels of oleic acid, a type of fat which has anti-inflammatory and heart health benefits.

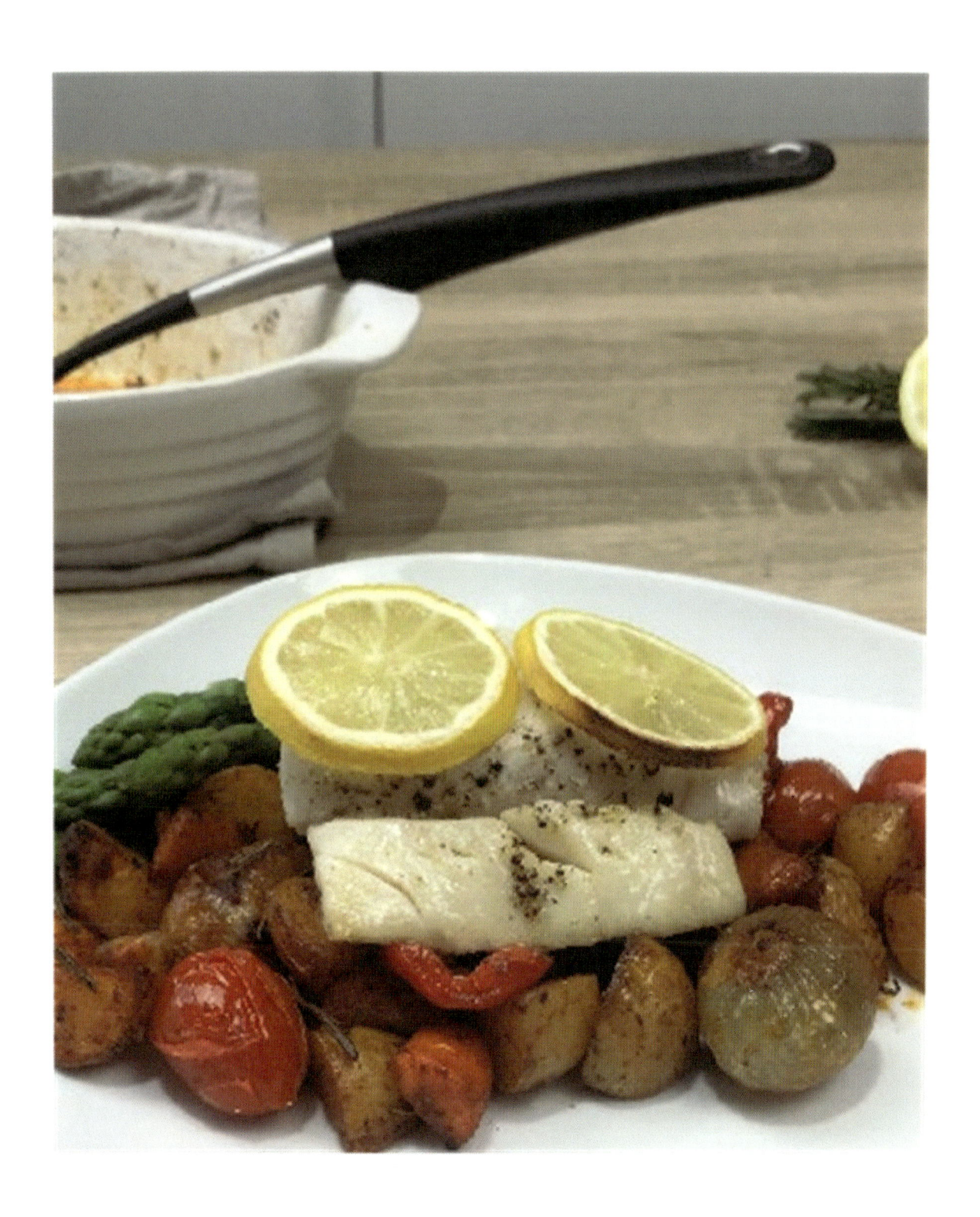

LAMB AND APRICOT TAGINE

(Per Serving) Calories 429 / Carbs 50g / Protein 28g / Fat 13g

Originating from Morocco and similar to a casserole, tagine is a satisfying, delicious one-pot wonder. Using a variety of aromatic spices creates a lovely depth of flavour that brings out the best in the lamb and apricots. Serve with rice and broccoli for a hearty dinner.

Serves 4 Prep Time 10 mins Cook Time 100 mins ## INGREDIENTS 1 ½ tbsp Olive Oil 600g (21 1/4oz) Diced Lamb 1 Large Onion 2 Garlic Cloves 200g (7oz) Carrot 400g (14oz) Tinned Chopped Tomatoes 1 tsp Cinnamon 1 tsp Turmeric 1 tsp Cumin 240g (8 1/2oz) Drained Chickpeas 1 Chicken Stock Cube 600ml (2 1/2cups) Boiling Water 80g (2 3/4oz) Apricots 200g (7oz) Broccoli 250g (8 3/4oz) Microwave Rice Optional: Coriander (cilantro) (roughly chopped)	## HOW TO COOK IT Preheat oven to 210°C. Add half the olive oil to a frying pan over a medium to high heat. When hot, add the lamb and brown the meat. Put the lamb to one side to rest while you prepare the rest of the meal. Add the remainder of the olive oil to the frying pan over a medium heat. Roughly chop the onion and, when the pan is hot, add the onion to the pan and cook for 5 minutes, or until the onions start to brown. Then finely chop the garlic and add to the pan for 1 minute. Peel the carrots, cut the ends off then quarter the carrots and put in the pan along with the tinned tomatoes, cinnamon, turmeric, cumin, drained chickpeas, chicken stock cube, boiling water and lastly the browned lamb meat. Stir all the ingredients together, cover with foil and place in the preheated oven for an hour. Chop the apricots, add to the casserole and stir before placing back in the oven for 30mins, without the tin foil. Meanwhile, prepare and cook the broccoli for 5 minutes and the rice for 2 minutes in the microwave. Serve. Optional extra - Chop up some coriander (cilantro) and sprinkle over the casserole.

DIETICIAN'S NOTES

Chickpeas and apricots are a great source of gut-friendly fibres - teamed with antioxidant rich spices, vegetables and wholegrain rice this is a nutrient dense meal.

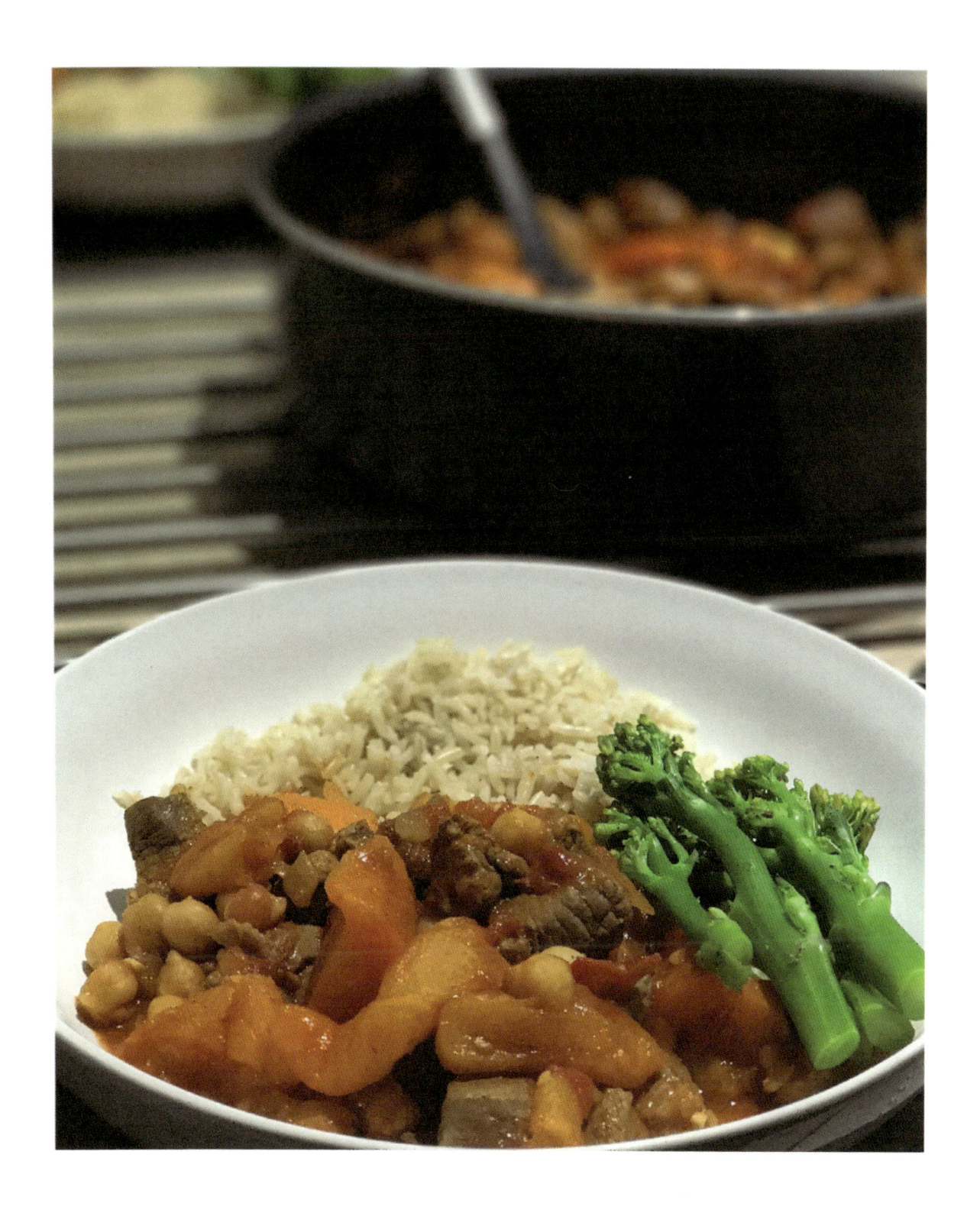

HEALTHY CHICKEN CURRY

(Per Serving) Calories 628 / Carbs 47g / Protein 47g / Fat 28g

Swap your take away for this deliciously healthy chicken curry. This twist on the classic recipe includes peas, cashew nuts and fresh coriander to make it stand out from the crowd. The Greek yogurt base keeps the calories down. Serve with coconut rice for extra flavour.

Serves 2 Prep Time 5 mins Cook Time 15 mins ## INGREDIENTS 1 tbsp Extra Virgin Olive Oil 250g (8 3/4oz) Chicken Breast ¾ Onion 1 Garlic Clove (finely chopped 1 tbsp Curry Powder 1 tsp Tomato Purée 3 tbsp Greek Yogurt 200ml (3/4cup) Chicken Stock Pinch of Salt and Pepper 300g (10 1/2oz) Coconut Grains (from Tesco) Or 250g Microwaveable Rice 25g (3/4oz) Cashew Nuts 75g (2 1/2oz) Frozen Peas 8 Sprigs Coriander (cilantro)	## HOW TO COOK IT Put half the olive oil in a pan over a medium heat. Cut the chicken into even-sized chunks and place in the frying pan. Do not cook through but part cook and then remove from the heat. To speed things up, in a separate pan, while the chicken is cooking, heat up the remainder of the olive oil. Finely chop the onion and place in the pan and cook until it starts to brown. As soon as the onion starts to brown, add the crushed up garlic and cook for 30 seconds. Then add the curry powder, tomato purée, Greek yogurt, chicken stock, salt, pepper and chicken into the pan, stir well and then leave to simmer on a low heat for 15 to 20 minutes or until the chicken is cooked through (don't leave the Greek yogurt in the pan for too long without stirring, otherwise it separates). Prepare your coconut grains in the microwave, as per the package instructions For the last 2 minutes, add the cashew nuts and peas to the curry and cook through. Plate up the coconut grains and curry, garnish with the coriander (cilantro) and serve. Note: If you can't get hold of the coconut grains, just use normal rice.

DIETICIAN'S NOTES

Adding peas to meals is a great way to boost your fibre intake, which helps protect against heart disease and bowel cancer. 100 grams peas = 20% of the recommended daily intake.

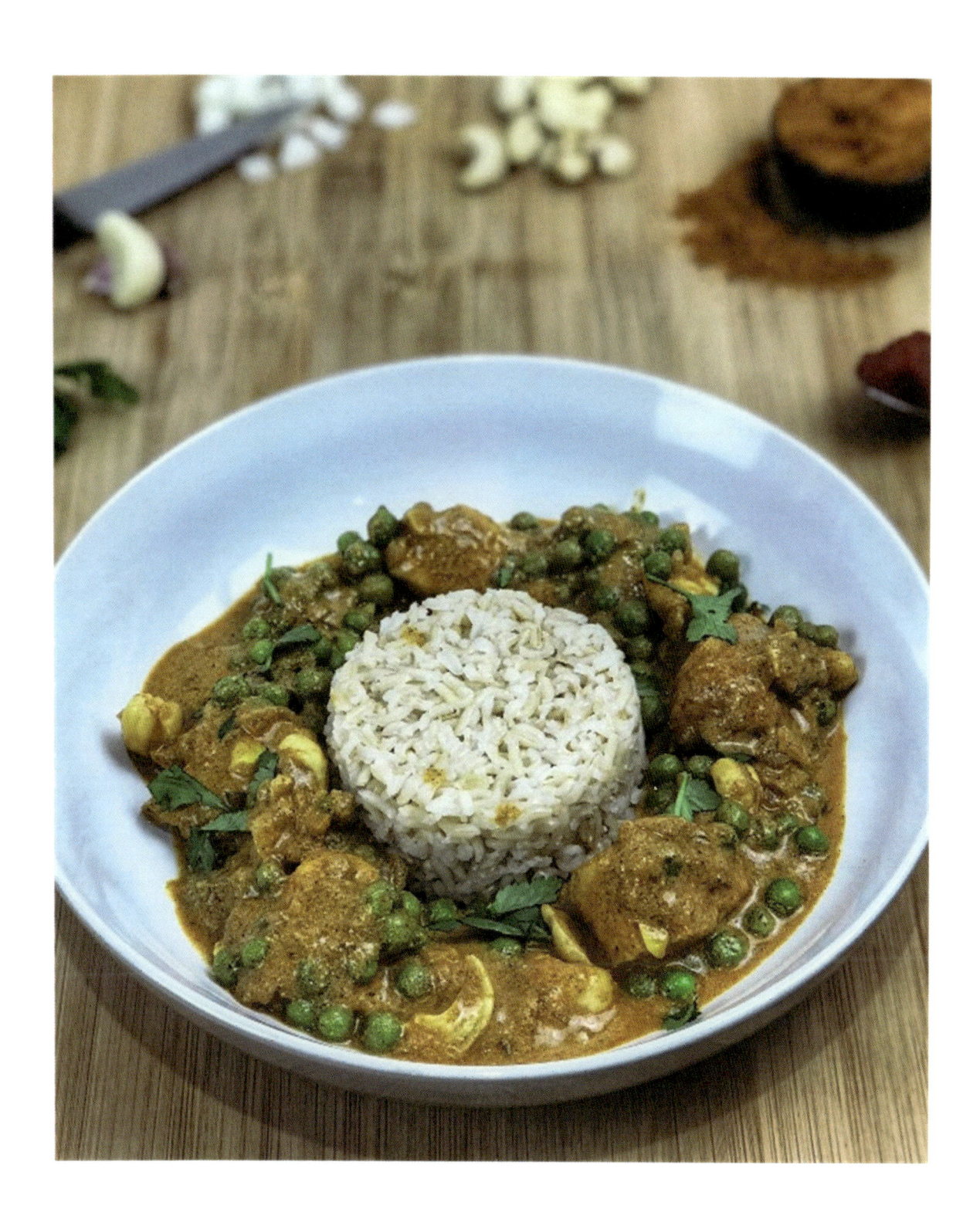

PAN FRIED SALMON ON A SALAD BED

(Per Serving) Calories 351 / Carbs 10g / Protein 35g / Fat 19g

Perfect for a weeknight dinner or weekday lunch, enjoy this flaky pan fried salmon served with a bed of ripe tomatoes, sweetcorn, cucumber and lettuce salad. A sweet balsamic dressing enhances the flavour of the salmon.

Serves 1 Prep Time 0 mins Cook Time 10 mins **INGREDIENTS** 1 tsp Extra Virgin Olive Oil 130g (4 1/2oz) Salmon 40g (1 1/2oz) Tomato 1/4 Cucumber 40g (1 1/2oz) Sweet Corn 2 x Lettuce Leaves (washed, dried & roughly chopped) 1 tsp Balsamic Vinegar Optional: Pinch of Salt & Pepper	**HOW TO COOK IT** Preheat ½ the olive oil in the frying pan on a medium heat. Add the salmon to the pan, skin side down and cook for roughly 3 minutes or until the skin is crisp. Turn the fish over and cook for a further 5 minutes. Then cook each side for 1 more minute. The fish is cooked when the salmon is nice and flakey. While the salmon is cooking, prepare your salad. Quarter the tomatoes. Peel, remove the seeds and slice the cucumber and drain the tinned sweetcorn. Add these to a mixing bowl along with the lettuce leaves. Add the remaining olive oil and balsamic vinegar to the mixing bowl and toss the salad and then plate up. When the salmon is cooked place it on top of the salad and enjoy! Optional: Add salt and pepper for flavour.

DIETICIAN'S NOTES

Eating salmon is a great way to top up your intake of omega-3 fats, which have anti inflammatory effects in the body. These essential fats can help with post workout muscle soreness.

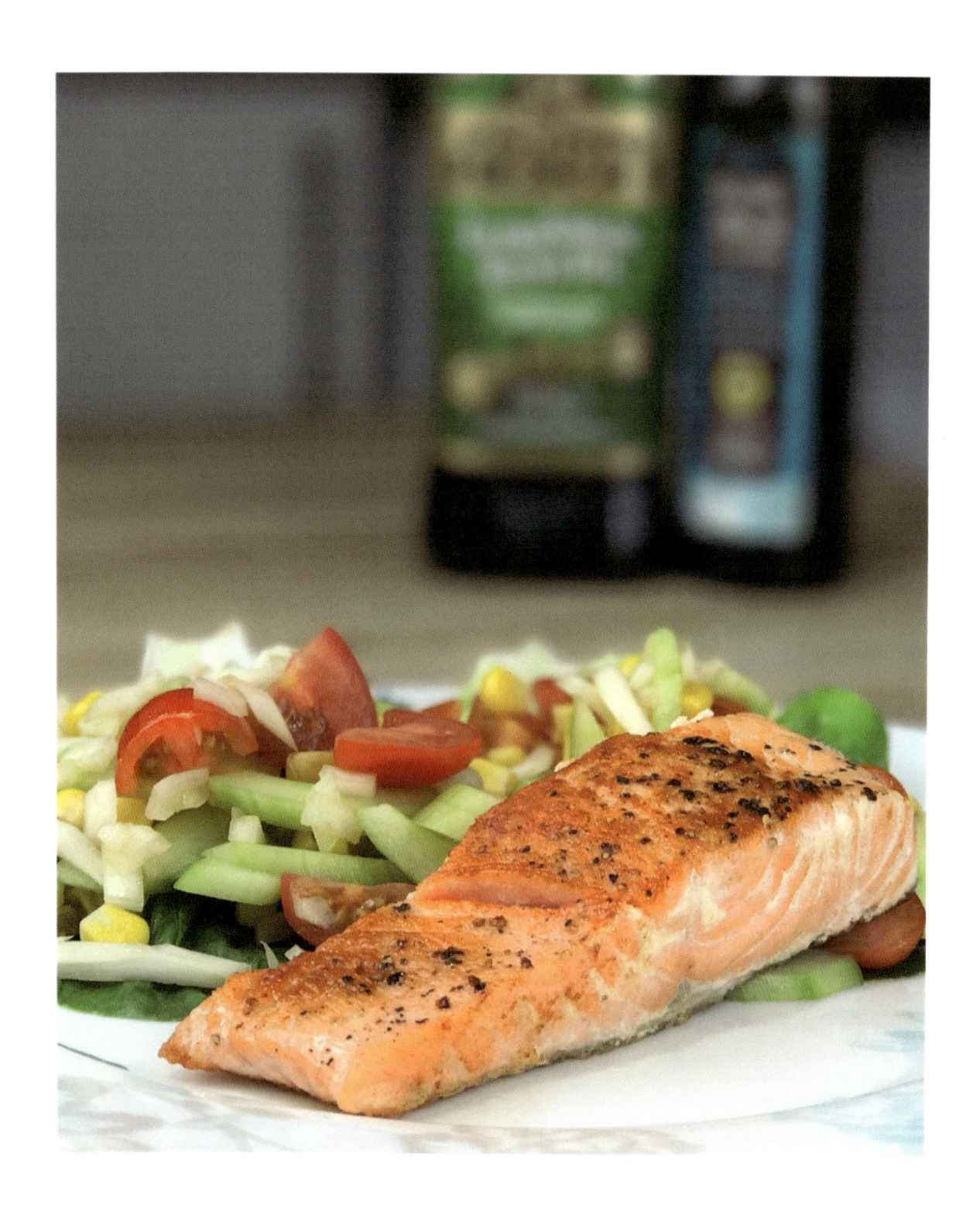

PARMA HAM WRAPPED CHICKEN WITH MOZZARELLA

(Per Serving) Calories 520 / Carbs 28g / Protein 57g / Fat 20g

This easy baked chicken will quickly become one of your favourite meals. The texture of the parma ham goes brilliantly with the tender chicken and the creamy mozzarella. Serve with new potatoes and broccoli.

Serves 2 Prep Time 10 mins Cook Time 40 mins ## INGREDIENTS 300g (10 1/2oz) New Potatoes (cut in half) 1 tbsp Olive Oil Pinch of Salt & Pepper 1 tsp Smoked Paprika 1 tsp Rosemary 2 x 150g (5 1/4oz) Chicken Breast 60g (2oz) Mozzarella (cut into slices) 6 Slices Parma Ham 100g (3 1/2oz) Broccoli 100g (3 1/2oz) Sugar Snap Peas	## HOW TO COOK IT Preheat oven to 200°C. Place the new potatoes in a bowl. Add the olive oil, salt, pepper, smoked paprika and rosemary to the new potatoes and mix. Spread the potatoes on a baking tray and place in the preheated oven for 40 minutes (you will add the chicken after 20 minutes). Meanwhile, create a slit down the side of the chicken breasts. Cut 4 slices of mozzarella and place 2 slices inside each chicken breast. Layout 3 pieces of Parma ham making sure they overlap and place the chicken in the center, then wrap the Parma ham around the chicken. Repeat with the other chicken breast. Place the chicken in the oven, along with the potatoes, for the last 20 minutes of cooking time. Cook the vegetables and serve up.

DIETICIAN'S NOTES

A protein packed dish, which should stave off hunger for a good few hours! Increase the portion size of the green vegetables for extra fibre - which helps nourish the good bacteria in your gut

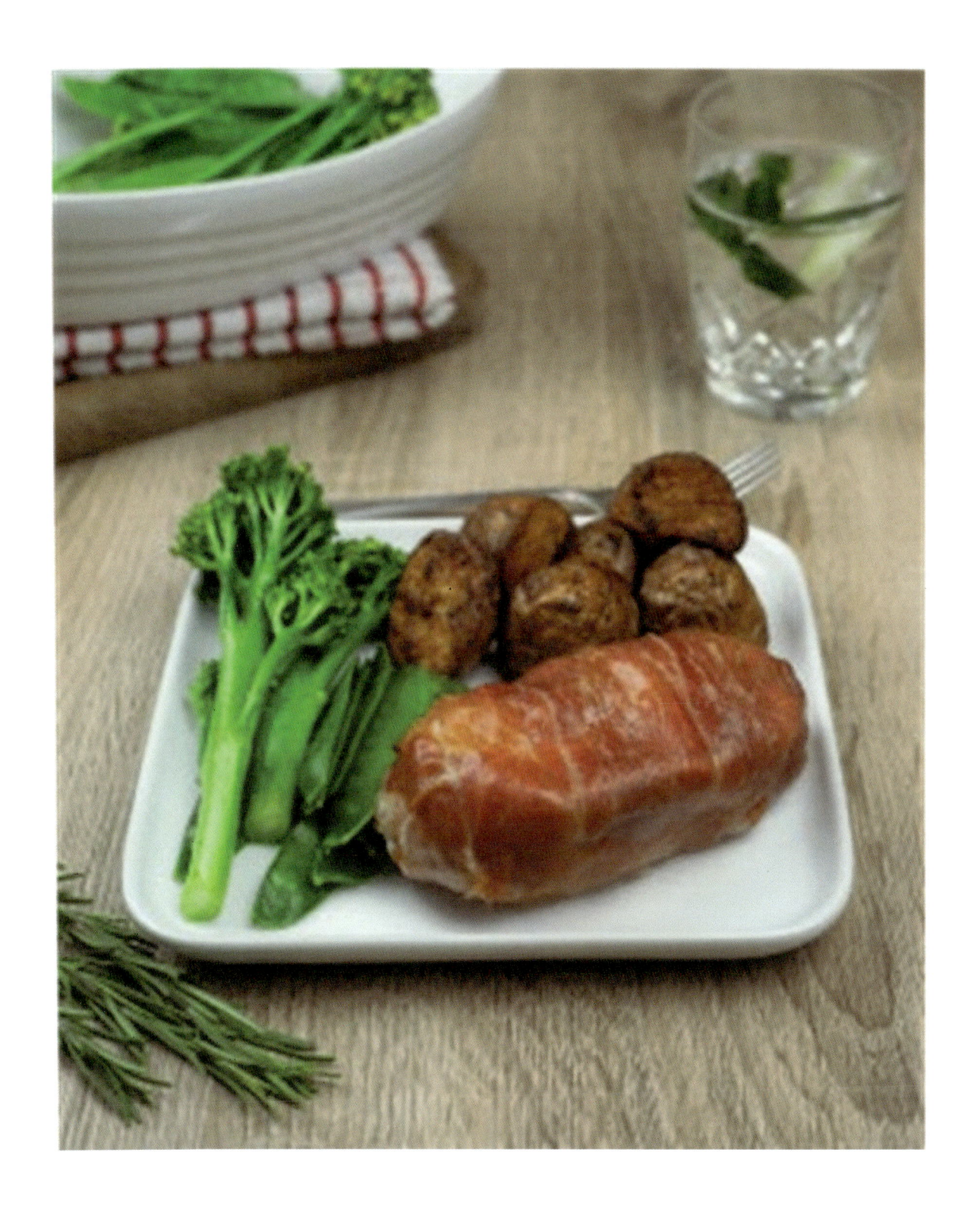

PRAWN AND CHORIZO PAELLA

(Per Serving) Calories 478 / Carbs 60g / Protein 37g / Fat 10g

Visit Spain without having to leave the house with this simple, quick paella recipe, which combines seafood, meat and colourful vegetables for a vibrant combination of flavours. This one-pan meal is packed with healthy ingredients - turmeric, roasted peppers, peas and juicy prawns. Viva la Espana!

Serves 2 Prep Time 5 mins Cook Time 22 mins ## INGREDIENTS 1 tsp Olive Oil ½ Red Onion (finely chopped) 1 Garlic Clove (finely chopped) 50g (1 3/4oz) Chorizo (roughly chopped) 125g (4 1/2oz) Paella Rice (dry weight) 1 Chicken Stock Cube 500ml (2cups) Boiling Water ¼ tsp Turmeric ¼ tsp Paprika 50g (1 3/4oz) Chopped Roasted Peppers 300g (10 1/2oz) Pre-Cooked Prawns (small shrimp) 100g (3 1/2oz) Frozen Peas Pinch Parsley (roughly chopped) ½ Lemon (cut in wedges)	## HOW TO COOK IT Heat the olive oil in a pan over a medium heat. Add the chopped onion, cook for 3 minutes. Add the chopped garlic and chorizo, cook for 2 minutes. Add the paella rice and stir. Dilute the chicken stock cube in the boiling water and add to the pan. Add the turmeric, paprika and chopped roasted peppers to the pan and stir. Simmer for 13 minutes, stirring occasionally. Add the cooked prawns (small shrimp) and peas, stir and cook for a further 4 minutes. Plate up, sprinkle the chopped parsley on top, squeeze the lemon over the dish and serve.

DIETICIAN'S NOTES

A great post-workout option containing carbohydrates to replenish energy levels, and protein, which supports muscle recovery and growth. Prawns (small shrimp) are also rich in selenium, which we need for immune function.

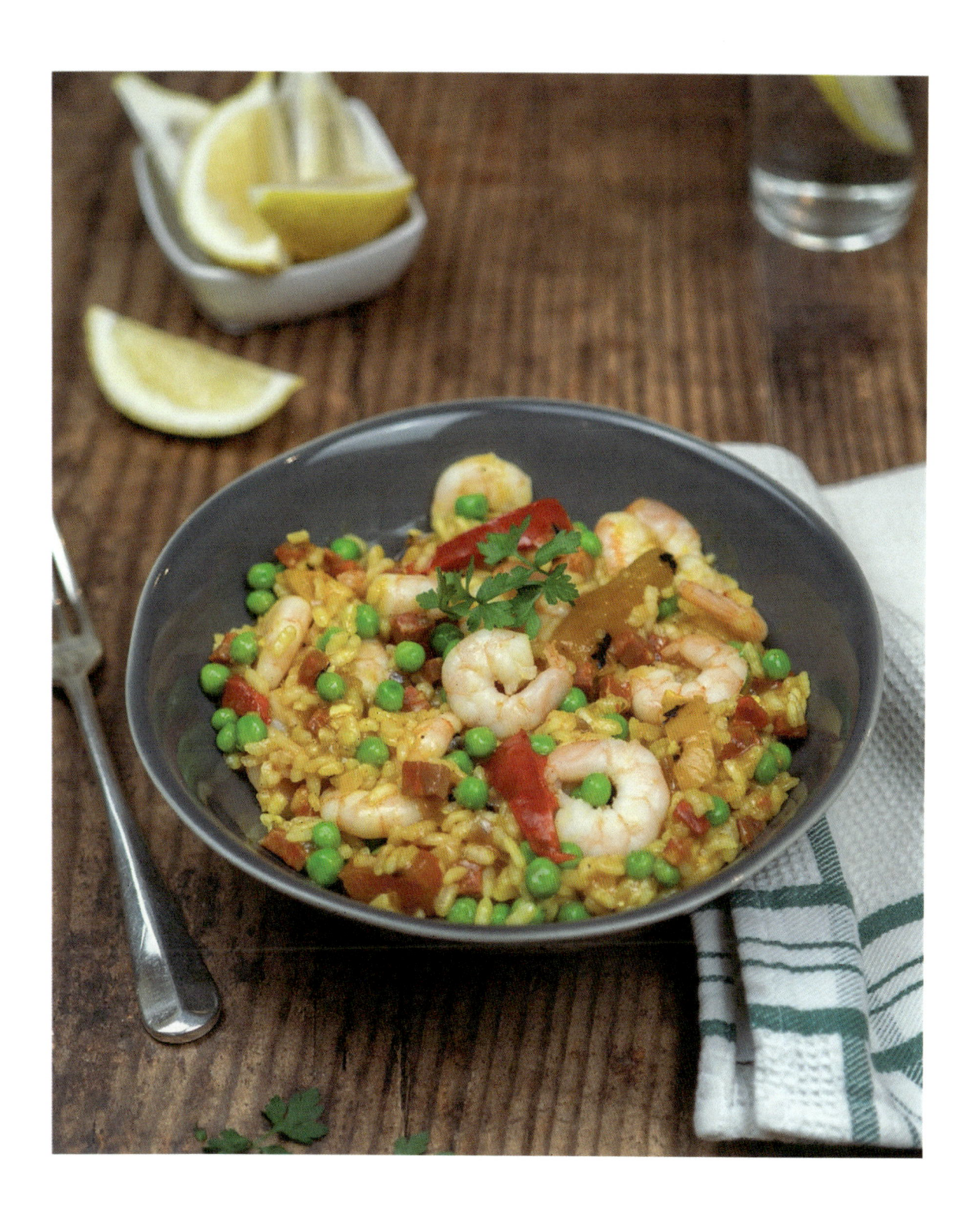

RED PEPPER AND CHICKEN TRAY BAKE

(Per Serving) Calories 620 / Carbs 34g / Protein 49g / Fat 32g

Indulge in this tasty one-pan roast chicken supper with lemon, cumin, paprika, coriander and other North African flavours. High in protein and low in saturated fat, this delicious traybake is a real mid-week lifesaver helping you save time and avoid stress.

Serves 2
Prep Time 10 mins Cook Time 40 mins

INGREDIENTS

1 tsp Lemon Zest
1 Lemon (Juiced)
1 tsp Smoked Paprika
½ tsp Cumin
½ tsp Fennel Seeds
3 tbsp Olive Oil
350g (12 1/4oz) Chicken Thighs (skinless & boneless)
250g (8 3/4oz) New Potatoes (cut into quaters)
100g (3 1/2oz) Onion
100g (3 1/2oz) Red Pepper
Salt & Pepper
100g (3 1/2oz) Broccoli
2 tbsp Greek Yogurt
Coriander (cilantro) (roughly chopped)

HOW TO COOK IT

Preheat oven to 200°C.

In a small mixing bowl add lemon zest, lemon juice, paprika, cumin, fennel seeds and olive oil. Mix it together and put to one side.

In a large mixing bowl, add skinless and boneless chicken thighs, new potatoes, onion and peppers.

Pour the mixture from the small mixing bowl in to the big mixing bowl, add salt and pepper and mix until all the chicken and vegetables are coated.

Put the mixture on to a baking tray and place in the preheated oven for 20 minutes.

Remove from the oven, stir and place back into the oven for a further 20 minutes.

Meanwhile, prepare the broccoli in boiling water (cook for between 3 and 5 minutes).

Plate up the food and add a tablespoon of Greek yogurt to each dish.

Sprinkle coriander (cilantro) over the top before serving.

Tip: Lower the calories and fat per serving by reducing the Olive Oil to 2 tbsp (instead of 3 tbsp). New Macros would be:
(Per Serving) Calories 559 / Carbs 34g / Protein 49g / Fat 25g

DIETICIAN'S NOTES

Using olive oil in cooking is a great habit - it's rich in monounsaturated fats, which are linked with a lower risk of heart disease. You'll also score two of your five-a-day with this dish.

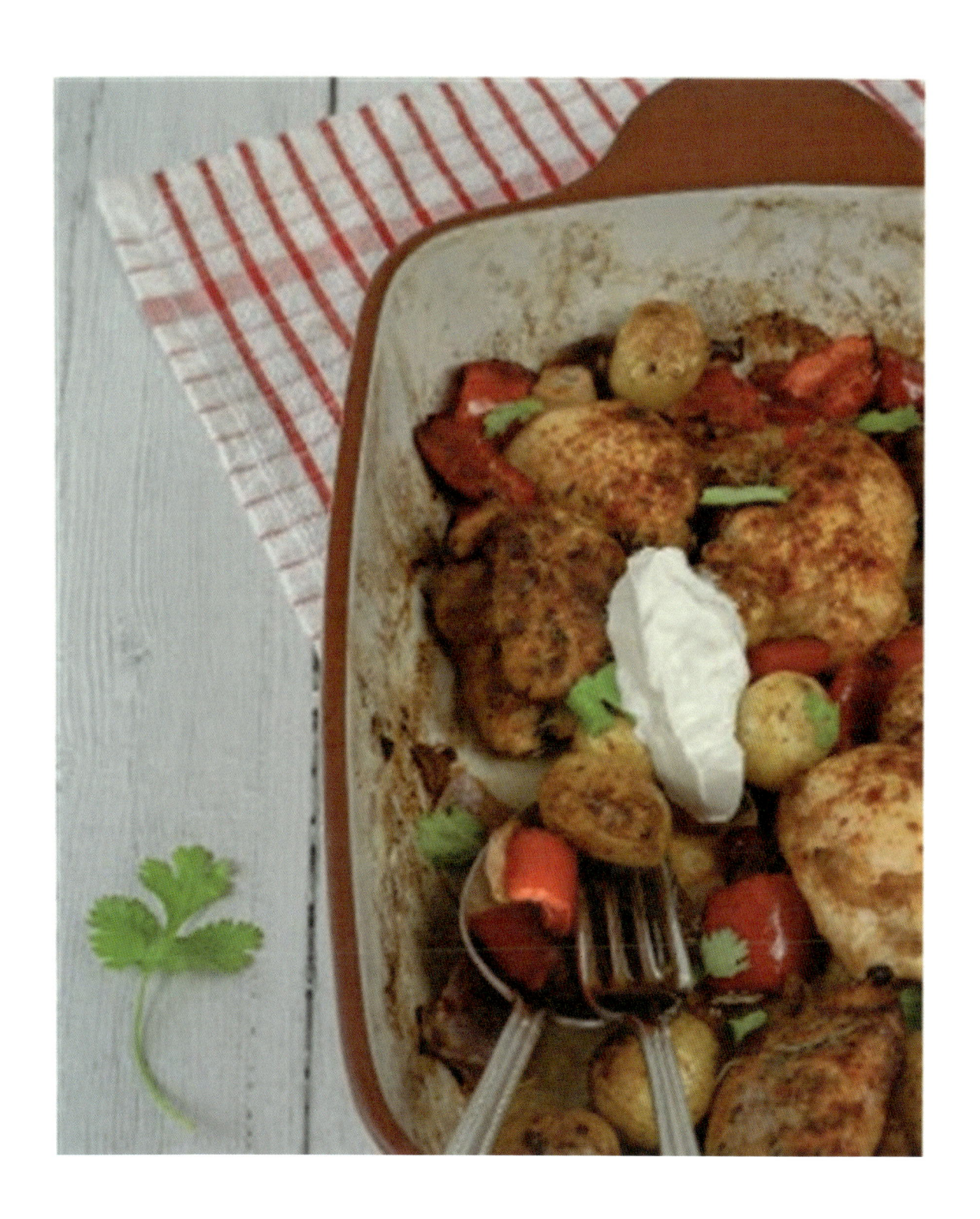

SALMON WITH GARLIC BUTTER HASSELBACK POTATOES

(Per Serving) Calories 490 / Carbs 32g / Protein 32g / Fat 26g

A great dish if you're having guests around! The baked salmon goes really well with the garlicky hasselback potatoes, which make for an impressive and tasty side dish. The potatoes are crispy on the outside and tender on the inside like the salmon. A sure-fire winner!

Serves 1 Prep Time 10 mins Cook Time 40 mins ## INGREDIENTS 200g (7oz) New Potatoes 15g (1/2oz) Butter 1 tsp Olive Oil 1 tsp Rosemary 1 Garlic Clove Salt & Pepper 130g (4 1/2oz) Salmon Fillet 100g (3 1/2oz) Vegetables or Side Salad	## HOW TO COOK IT Preheat oven to 200°C. Part slice the top of the potatoes several times and place on a baking tray. Melt the butter in the microwave, mix in the olive oil, rosemary, finely chopped garlic, salt and pepper and stir. Brush half the mixture over the potatoes and put in the preheated oven for 20 mins. Remove the potatoes from the oven and place the salmon on the baking tray with them. Sprinkle a little salt and pepper over the salmon and the brush some of the butter mixture onto the salmon. Brush the remainder of the butter mixture onto the potatoes and cook for a further 20mins. With 5 minutes to go, prepare your chosen vegetables. Serve up and enjoy!

DIETICIAN'S NOTES

Omega-3 fats in salmon (& other oily fish) help protect against low mood & depression. Two portions of oily fish per week can also reduce your risk of heart disease - tick off one portion with this dish.

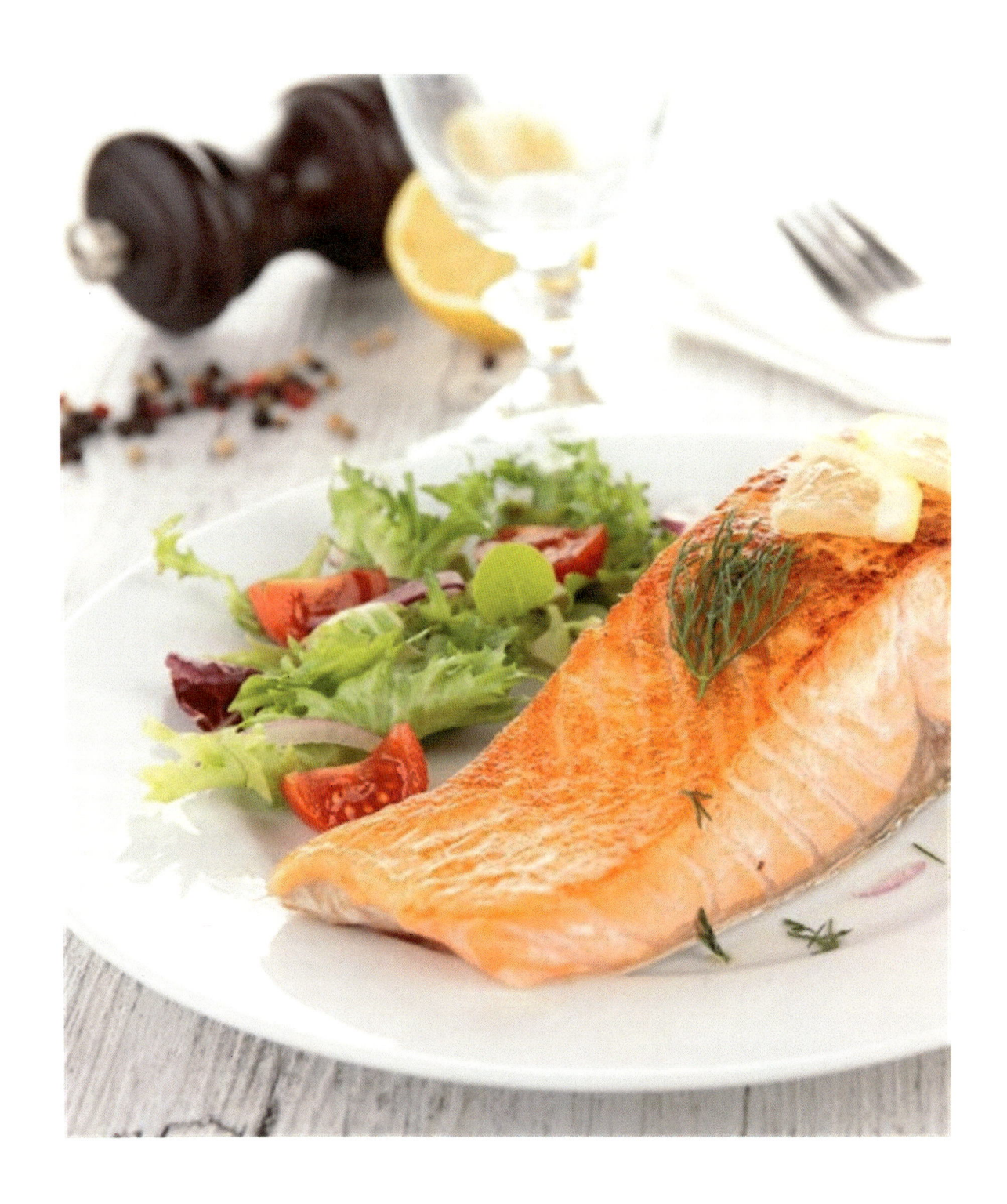

TURKEY MEATBALLS IN TOMATO SAUCE

(Per Serving) Calories 544 / Carbs 50g / Protein 41g / Fat 20g

Light, succulent and low in fat, these tender meatballs are ready in less than thirty minutes for an easy midweek meal. Replacing beef with turkey meat creates a leaner, healthier dish which doesn't affect the delicious, classic, rich flavours.

Serves 2 Prep Time 5 mins Cook Time 20 mins ## INGREDIENTS 2 tsp Extra Virgin Olive Oil 400g (14oz) Turkey Mince ½ Onion 1 Garlic Clove 400g (14oz) Can of Tinned Tomatoes Salt & Pepper Pinch of Dried Rosemary Pinch of Dried Mixed Herbs Pinch of Dried Oregano 4 x 50g (1 3/4oz) Vegetable 250g (8 3/4oz) Microwavable Brown Rice	## HOW TO COOK IT Heat 1 tsp of olive oil in a frying pan on a medium to high heat. If using pre-made turkey meatballs, place them into the pan and brown all the sides. If making from scratch, roll the turkey mince into balls then place them into the pan and brown them off. Once done, place the meatballs to one side. Heat a tsp of olive oil in a large frying pan on a medium heat. Peel and finely chop the onion, place into the pan and cook until the onion starts to brown. Peel and finely chop the garlic and place into the pan, cook for 30 seconds. Add the meatballs back into the pan along with the tinned tomatoes, salt and pepper, dried rosemary, dried mixed herbs and dried oregano and stir well. Cook for 15 minutes stirring occasionally. While the meatballs are cooking, heat a pan with water and cook your chosen vegetables and microwave your rice. Serve everything up and enjoy!

DIETICIAN'S NOTES

A great option for a post workout meal - tomatoes are rich in lycopene, an antioxidant shown to help with muscle

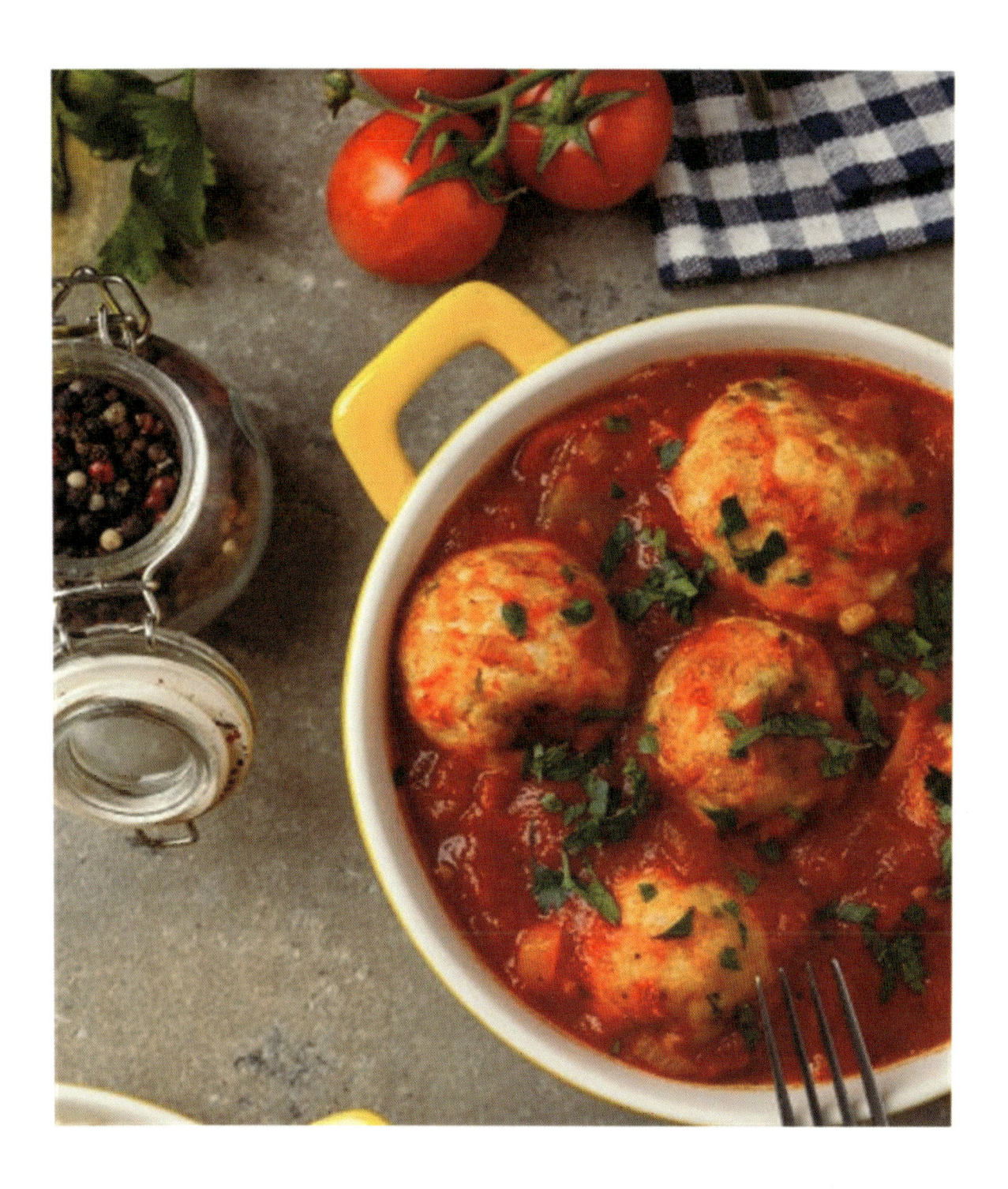

CHICKEN TIKKA KEBABS

(Per Serving) Calories 432 / Carbs 45g / Protein 45g / Fat 8g

We've given kebabs a makeover! Marinate tender chicken breasts and cook with crunchy onions, juicy tomatoes and sweet peppers. Serve with a side of sweet potato fries and salad for a speedy mid-week meal.

Serves 2
Prep Time 15 mins Cook Time 40 mins

INGREDIENTS

300g (10 1/2oz) Sweet Potato (Halve and cut into thin chips)
2 tsp Olive Oil
Pinch of Salt & Pepper
1 tsp Paprika
1 tsp Rosemary
300g (10 1/2oz) Chicken Breast
1 tbsp Tikka Powder
120g (4 1/4oz) Greek Yogurt
1 ½ Coloured Peppers (cut into cubes)
½ Red Onion (cut into squares)
6 Baby Tomatoes
1 tsp Mint
30g (1oz) Cucumber (peel, cut in half and remove the middle of the cucumber with a spoon)
60g (2oz) Rocket Leaves
1 tsp Balsamic Vinegar

HOW TO COOK IT

Preheat oven to 200°C (392°F).

Place the sweet potatoes into a large mixing bowl.

Add 1 tsp of olive oil to the chips as well as salt, pepper, paprika and rosemary and mix well so all the chips are covered.

Put the chips on to a baking tray and then place in the preheated oven for 40 minutes (flip them over after 20 minutes, when you start cooking the kebabs).

Cut the chicken breasts into chunks and add to a mixing bowl.

Add the tikka powder and 70g Greek yogurt and mix well.

If you have time, marinate in the fridge for a few hours for more flavour.

In a random order, place the chicken pieces, onion, pepper and tomatoes onto the kebab skewers.

Place the kebab skewers in the oven for the last 20 minutes with the sweet potato chips.

In a small mixing bowl, add 50g Greek yogurt and dried mint. Then cut the cucumber into small pieces, add to small mixing bowl and mix well.

Divide the rocket leaves between 2 plates, and then add the chicken and vegetables from each kebab skewer to the plates.

Mix 1 tsp of olive oil and 1 tsp of balsamic vinegar together and pour over the salads before serving.

DIETICIAN'S NOTES

A colourful meal packed with antioxidants that support your body's immune system. The balance of protein and carbohydrates would make this a great post-workout meal.

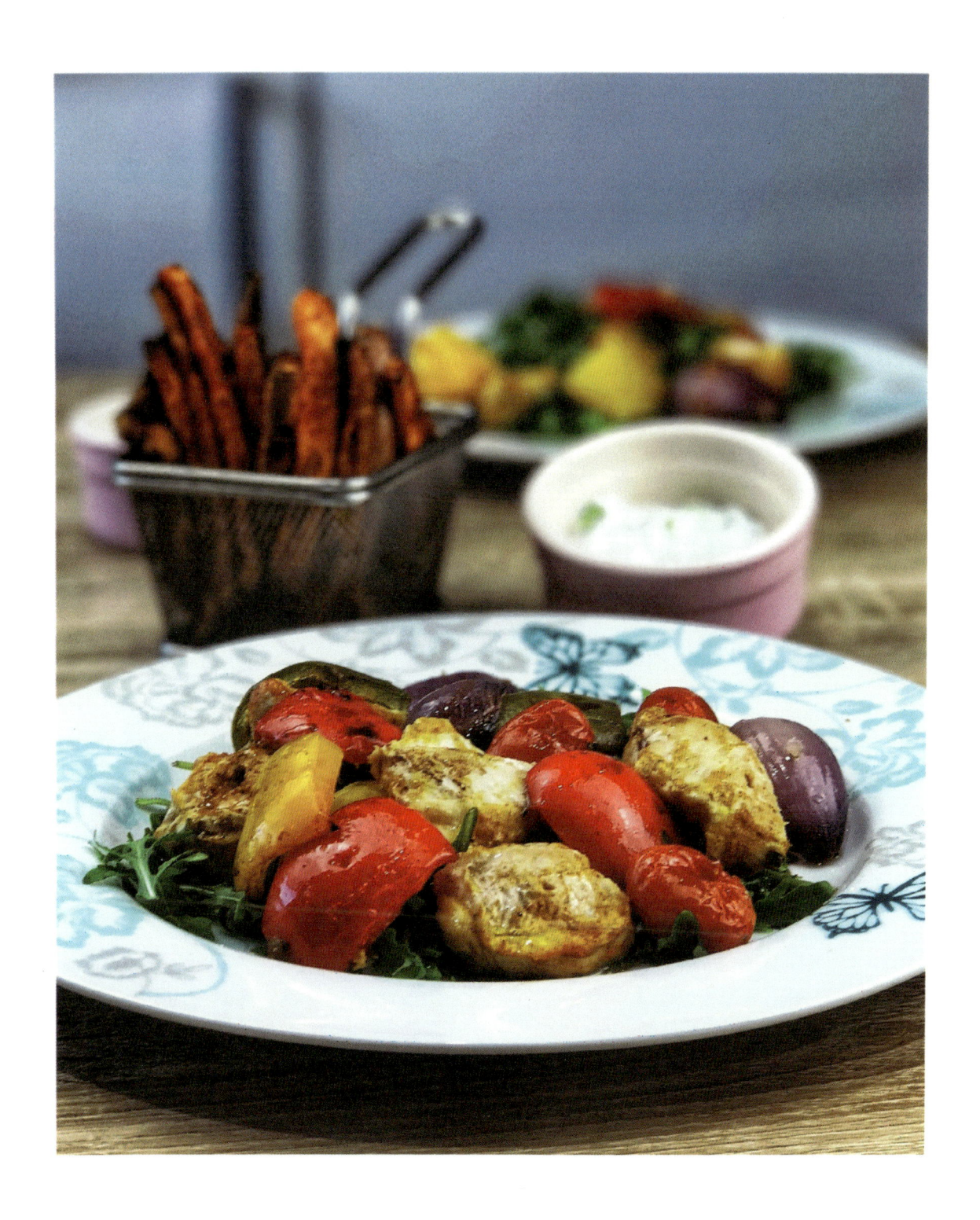

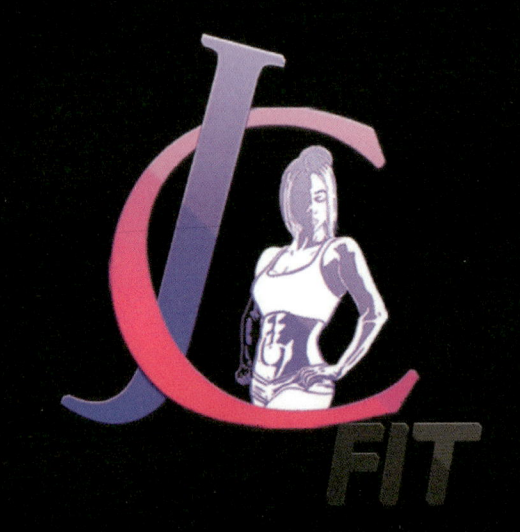

Printed in Great Britain
by Amazon